STUDENT WORKBOOK
for
PRACTICE MANAGEMENT
for the
DENTAL TEAM

7th Edition

STUDENT WORKBOOK
for
PRACTICE MANAGEMENT
for the
DENTAL TEAM

7th Edition

Betty Ladley Finkbeiner, CDA Emeritus, BS, MS
Emeritus Faculty
Washtenaw Community College
Ann Arbor, Michigan

Charles Allan Finkbeiner, BS, MS
Emeritus Faculty
Washtenaw Community College
Ann Arbor, Michigan

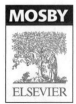

MOSBY

ELSEVIER

3251 Riverport Lane
St. Louis, Missouri 63043

STUDENT WORKBOOK FOR PRACTICE MANAGEMENT   ISBN: 978-0-323-06535-1
FOR THE DENTAL TEAM

ISBN: 978-0-323-06535-1

Vice President and Publisher: Linda Duncan
Executive Editor: John Dolan
Managing Editor: Kristin Hebberd
Publishing Services Manager: Julie Eddy
Project Manager: Marquita Parker
Designer: Charlie Seibel

Printed in United States

Last digit is the print number: 9   8   7   6   5

Working together to grow
libraries in developing countries

www.elsevier.com | www.bookaid.org | www.sabre.org

ELSEVIER   BOOK AID International   Sabre Foundation

Introduction to the Student

The Student Workbook, CD-ROM, and Patterson EagleSoft practice management software have been integrated to help you practice and perfect the skills and objectives emphasized in *Practice Management for the Dental Team,* 7th Edition. The Student Workbook includes the following information, exercises, and activities to help you succeed within the office environment and become a valuable member of the dental team:

- **Chapter Summaries** briefly recap the key concepts and goals of each chapter.
- **Learning Outcomes** identify the knowledge and skills necessary to master the topic areas discussed in each chapter.
- **Short-Answer or Fill-In Questions** help you to identify and list information from knowledge learned in the chapter as well as learn to apply that information to real-world practice in a dental office environment. Some of the questions also require you to synthesize the information and decide how you might handle certain situations in a practice environment.
- **Multiple-Choice Questions** and **Matching Exercises** ask you to recall information and concepts presented within the chapter and in some instances to think critically and apply the information to achieve best practice and professional success.
- **Practical Activities** put you, the student, into the role of the practicing professional and ask you to complete realistic daily tasks, pulling information learned within the chapters and putting that into practice.
- **Software Tutorials** introduce you to real-world dental practice in the form of the Patterson EagleSoft practice management software program. The tutorials direct you step by step through a series of exercises that demonstrate basic and advanced functions typically performed in day-to-day dental office management. Tutorials are included for Chapter 7 on patient information and dental office documents, Chapter 11 on appointment scheduling and management, Chapter 12 on recall procedures, Chapter 14 on dental insurance, and Chapter 15 on accounts receivable. Tutorial skills progress throughout these chapters, and it is important to complete them in the chapter order in which they are presented to maximize their effectiveness.
- **Critical Thinking Activities** pose potential situations and ask you to use what you have learned to determine how best they can be handled to achieve success in the office environment.
- **Internet Assignments** encourage you to perform website searches to gain a broader knowledge of the wide level of information available online and to learn to perform simple research that can improve your performance as a member of the dental team.

We hope that the information included throughout this entire learning package provides you with the confidence and skills needed to achieve long-term career success!

Betty Ladley Finkbeiner
Charles Allan Finkbeiner

Contents

How to Use Patterson Eaglesoft Practice Management Software

Each copy of *Practice Management for the Dental Team* is packaged with a complimentary copy of Patterson EagleSoft.

This is a demonstration version of the EagleSoft program that *must be installed onto your computer* in order to work. This demonstration version allows you to explore and become familiar with the program, as well as work through the Software Tutorial sections found in workbook Chapters 7, 11, 12, 14, and 15. Additional practice exercises are available on the Evolve website.

Before attempting to install this program on a computer in a school's computer lab facility, please discuss with your instructor or administrator to check on your school's installation policy.

SYSTEM REQUIREMENTS

Pentium IV or higher
1 GB of RAM or better
20× or higher CD-ROM drive
1024 × 768, 32 bit (thousands of colors) color display or better
500 MB available hard disk free-space
Printer available to print "Help" topics or documentation as needed
Windows® Server 2003, Windows® XP Professional, or Windows Vista Business, Ultimate or Enterprise

INSTALLATION

For technical support regarding the **installation** of this program, contact EagleSoft at 800-475-5036 and provide reference name *Elsevier*. When calling the Patterson Technology Center, please indicate to the receptionist that you are a student using the *Student Workbook for Practice Management for the Dental Team*. For assistance with exercises or functions of this program, please consult your instructor.

Before you begin, following is a listing of four known issues with installation, none of which should hinder your use of the EagleSoft program:

1. *Uninstalling program changes system font:* In Windows Vista and Windows 7, when the program was uninstalled, the default system font "Segoe UI" was removed from the Windows Font directory. As a result, the default system font was changed to "Segoe UI Italic."
2. *Uninstalling leaves files on system:* In Windows Vista and Windows 7, the following files were left on the system after uninstalling the program:
       C:\EagleSoft Autobackups\<date>\EagleSoft\Data\dental.db
       C:\EagleSoft Autobackups\<date>\EagleSoft\Data\dental.log
   In Windows XP Pro, a zip file was left on the system after uninstalling the program:
       C:\EagleSoft Autobackups\<date>.zip
   This contained the folder EagleSoft\Data with the files dental.dll and dental.txt.
3. *Installer launches internal update:* In Windows XP Pro, when launching and logging into EagleSoft, an internal update runs. When this completes, a message box with no message text pops up. This box will close when the user hits *OK*.
4. *Installer changes system folder options:* In Windows XP Pro, when the CD-ROM auto-run launcher started, the text below Explorer icons was changed to active links. In order to restore the default setting, go into *Folder Options → General* and change the *Click items as follows* option back to the default. Double-click to open an item (single-click to select).

Insert the Patterson EagleSoft demonstration disk into your computer's CD-ROM drive. If you have enabled your system's Auto-Start function, the Demonstration window appears automatically and you can skip to Step 5 below. If the start-up wizard does not appear automatically, you must complete Steps 1-4 below.

1. Close all software applications on your computer, including Windows Explorer.
2. Select *Run* from the Windows Start Menu. The Run window appears.
3. Type "D:\runme.exe" in the open field. (If the CD-ROM drive on your computer is represented by a different letter for the drive, substitute the appropriate letter for "D").

How to Use Patterson Eaglesoft Practice Management Software

4. The EagleSoft Demonstration window appears. Select *Software Installation*.

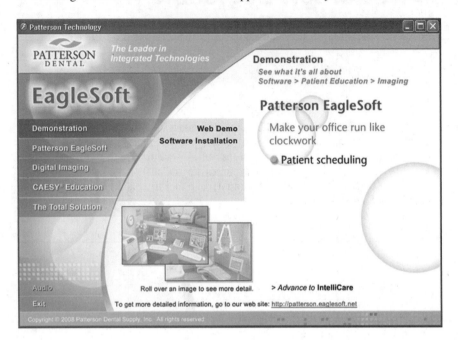

5. To review the Installation instructions, select *Click here to view installation instructions*.

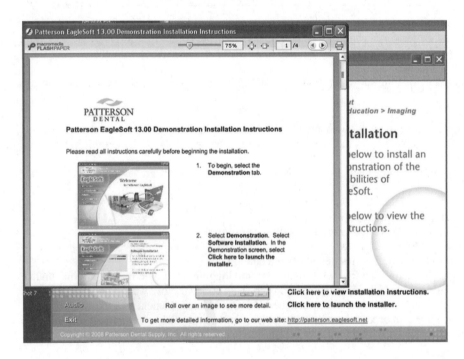

6. The Welcome window appears. Select *Next*.

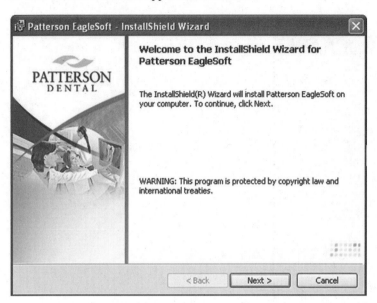

7. Read the License Agreement. If you agree to the terms, click the radio button next to the sentence *I accept the terms in the license agreement*. Then select *Next*.

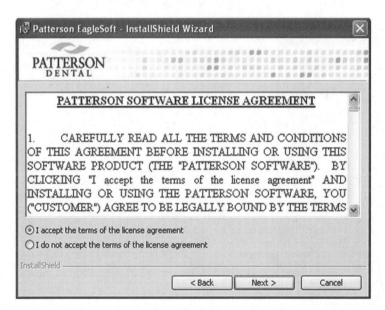

The demonstration CD *is not* compatible with Windows XP Home Edition and will not install on such systems. The EagleSoft program is intended for professional use.

How to Use Patterson Eaglesoft Practice Management Software

8. You will then see a screen requesting a license number. Please leave the spaces blank and simply select *Next* to advance.

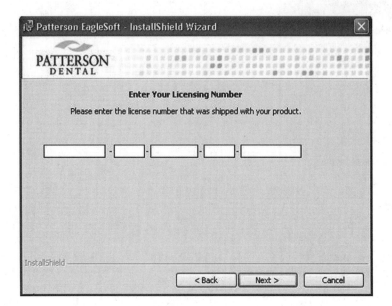

9. The InstallShield Wizard window will appear near; select *Install*.

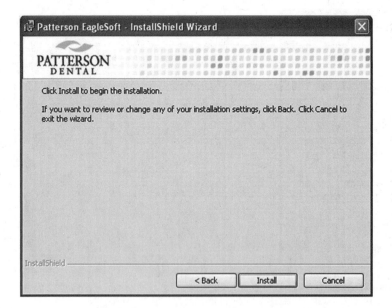

10. When the installation is completed, select *Finish* in the InstallWizard Completed window.

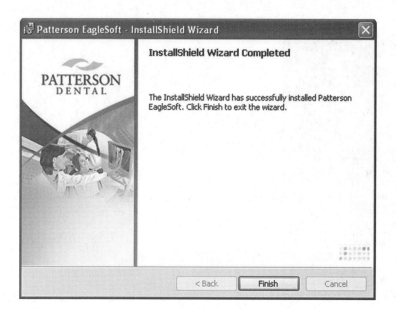

11. Select *OK* to restart your computer.

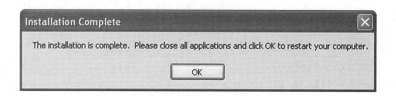

12. You can now remove the disk from the CD drive. It is not necessary to reinsert the disk each time you use the Patterson EagleSoft program.

USING THE PATTERSON EAGLESOFT DEMONSTRATION PROGRAM

How to Log In

1. Click on the Patterson EagleSoft desktop icon, or select *Start → Programs → EagleSoft → Patterson EagleSoft*.
2. A window appears notifying you that this is a demonstration version. Select *OK*.

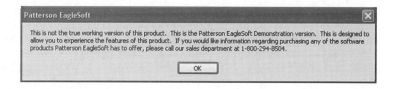

3. The Logon window appears next. Select *James Patton* from the provider drop-down list box. A password is not needed in the Password field. Select *Logon*.

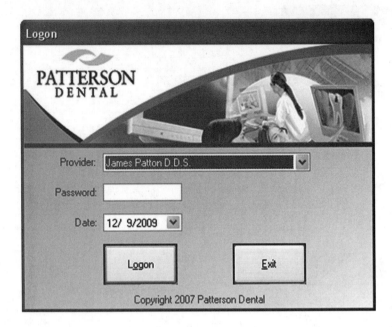

Keyboard Shortcuts

Shortcut	Function
Ctrl key + P	Opens Person List window
Ctrl key + W	Opens Walkout Processing window
Ctrl + Shift +P	Opens Receive Payments window
F1 key	Opens the Online User's Guide
F5 key	Recalls the last patient in the system
F2 key	Opens List windows in various screens

Viewing Modes

The program opens in the Integrated Mode. To view the Practice Management Mode, select *Window → Practice Management Mode*. To view the Clinical Mode, select *Window → Clinical Mode*.

NOTE: The software exercises in the workbook utilize the EagleSoft demonstration program in the Practice Management Mode or Integrated Mode. The Practice Management Mode is shown below:

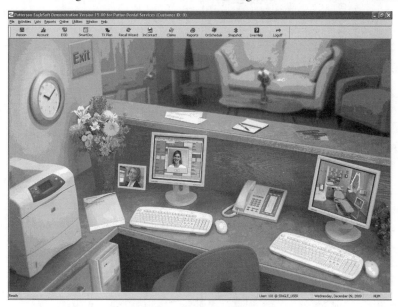

Viewing and Editing Practice Information

Only information on the Messages, Notes, and Preferences tabs can be edited.

1. From the Lists menu, select *Practice Information*. The Practice Information window appears, as shown below:

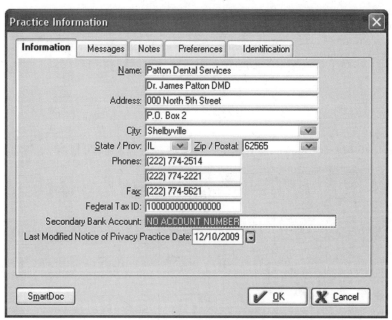

2. Select the *Messages, Notes,* or *Preferences* tabs to edit any information.
3. Select *OK* to save and exit the Practice Information window.

Viewing and Editing Providers

All information can be edited.

1. From the Lists menu, select *Providers/Staff*.
2. Select a provider and select *Edit*.

How to Use Patterson Eaglesoft Practice Management Software

3. The Edit Provider/Staff window appears.

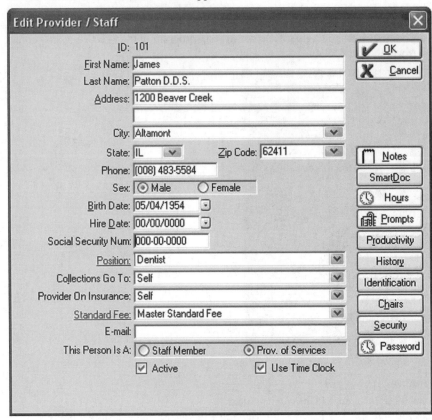

4. If desired, edit any of the information in the fields or drop-down list boxes.
5. The toolbar on the right side of the window offers methods of editing information, such as adding notes, changing hours, editing prompts, viewing productivity, and more.
6. Select *OK* to save and exit the Edit Provider/Staff window.
7. Select *Close* on the Provider/Staff window.

Viewing and Editing Patients

All information can be edited.
1. From the Lists menu, select *Person*.
2. Select a person from the Person List. Select *Edit* once a person is selected.
3. If desired, edit any of the information in the fields or drop-down list boxes.

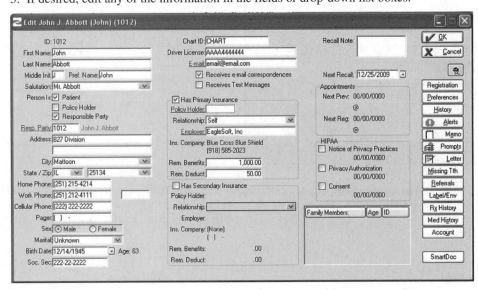

4. The toolbar on the right side of the window offers methods of editing information, such as adding preferences or alerts; viewing patient, medical and prescription history; and entering prompts, referrals and missing teeth.
5. Select *OK* to save and exit the Edit Person window.
6. Select *Close* on the Person List window.

Attaching an Insurance Company to a Policy Holder

1. From the Lists menu, select *Person.*
2. Select a person from the Person List. Select *Edit* once a person is selected.
3. If it is not selected, select the *Policy Holder* check box. The Policy Holder, Relationship, Employer, Remaining Benefits and Remaining Deductible fields are now available.
4. Select the checkbox next to *Has Primary Insurance* or *Has Secondary Insurance.* The Policy Holder Number appears and Self appears in the Relationship field.
5. To assign an employer to the patient, select in the *Employer* field and press the *F2* key, or select the underlined word Employer. The Employer List window appears.
6. Select the patient's employer (the insurance company appears next to the employer name) and select *Use.* The employer and insurance information appears with the remaining benefits and deductible.
7. A message will appear asking "Do you want to update the employer information?" Select *Yes* to save and exit.
8. From the Person List window, select *Close.*

Attaching an Insurance Company to a Dependent

1. From the Lists menu, select *Person.*
2. Select a person from the Person List. Select *Edit* once a person is selected.

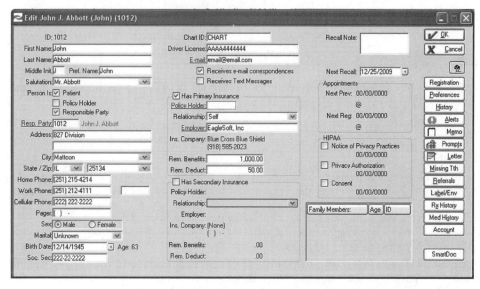

3. If it is not selected, select the *Has Primary Insurance* or *Has Secondary Insurance* check box. The Policy Holder, Relationship, Employer, Remaining Benefits and Remaining Deductible fields are now available.
4. Select in the *Policy Holder* field and press the *F2* key, or select the underlined words Policy Holder. The Policy Holder List window appears. Select the policy holder for this patient and select *Use.* Once this is done, a Policy Holder Number appears, the type of the relationship appears in the Relationship field (use the drop-down list to select a relationship) and the policyholder's employer appears. If the employer's insurance information has been entered, the insurance company appears below the Employer field.
5. Select *OK* to save and exit.
6. From the Person List window, select *Close.*

Scheduling Daily Appointments

1. From the Practice Management toolbar, select the *OnSchedule* button. The OnSchedule window appears.
2. Right-click in the white area. A menu appears with scheduling options.
3. Choose *Schedule Appointment* from the menu. A Patient List window appears.
4. Select a patient from the Patient List window and select *Use.*
5. The New Appointment window appears for the selected patient (see p. xviii). Patient and account information appears in the top portion of the window. If desired, you can change the appointment type, provider, or time units and enter a prefix, amount, or notes.

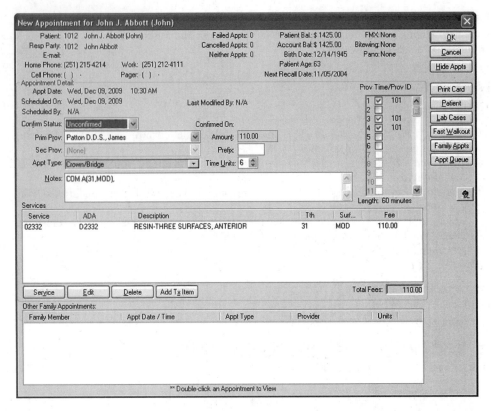

6. Select *Service* to attach a service to this appointment according to the Service or ADA Code, Service Type and Description.
7. Highlight the service and select the *Use* button.
8. Select *OK* to enter the appointment.

Processing a Walkout Statement

1. From the toolbar, select the *Walkout* button. The Walkout Statement window appears.
2. Select the *Patient* field and press the *F2* key to access the Person List window. You can also select the Patient hyperlink.
3. Select a patient and then select *Use*. The patient's information appears in the top portion of the Walkout Statement window. If this patient has a treatment plan, please follow the remaining instructions in this step. If not, proceed to the next step.
   a. A window appears with the following message: "This patient has planned/scheduled procedures. Do you want to select items to be completed?" Select *Yes* to select treatment plan items.
   b. From the Treatment Plan Items window, select the items you want to include on the walkout and Select the *Mark* button. To include all items, select the *Mark All* button.
   c. When finished selecting items, select *OK*. The selected items will appear in the Walkout Statement window.
4. The blinking cursor appears in the Service field. To add services to the walkout statement, press the *F2* key to access the Service Codes List window.
5. Select the *Service Code* radio button to sort the list by the service code.
6. Select a service and select *Use*.
7. Repeat steps 4 through 6 if you wish to add more services to the walkout statement.
8. Select *Process* once you are ready to begin processing this walkout statement. The Walkout Processing window appears (see p. xix).

How to Use Patterson Eaglesoft Practice Management Software

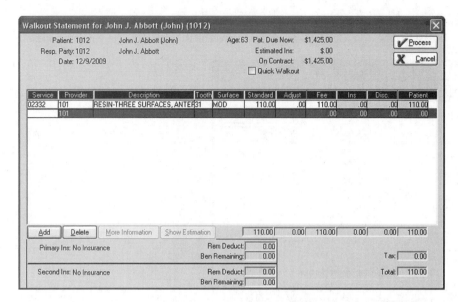

9. From the Walkout Processing window, enter a payment on the walkout or a credit adjustment on the account by entering the payments or credit adjustments in their fields. Select *OK*.
10. A window appears asking if you are ready to process this walkout statement. Select *Yes*.
11. If there is insurance on this walkout, the Insurance Questions window appears. Select the *Print Now* radio button. Select *OK* to print the insurance claim and to finish processing the walkout.

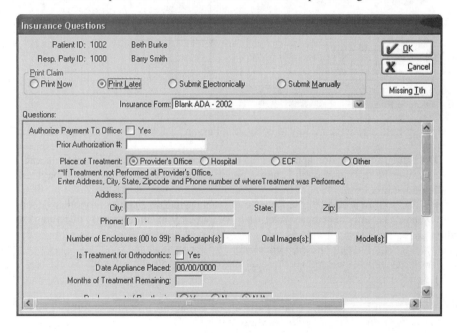

How to Use Patterson Eaglesoft Practice Management Software

Posting Payments

1. From the Practice Management toolbar, select the *Acct (Account) Payment* button. The Receive Payment window appears.

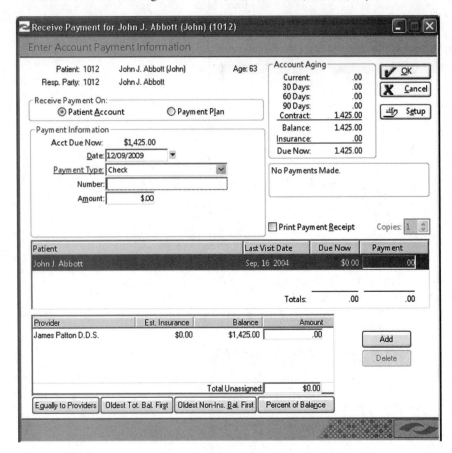

2. The blinking cursor appears in the Patient field. Press the *F2* key to access the Person List window. You can also select the underlined word <u>Patient</u>.
3. Select a patient and then select *Use*. The patient's information appears in the top portion of the Receive Payment window.
4. The blinking cursor appears in the Number field. If applicable, enter a check number, or select a different payment type from the Payment Type drop-down list box.
5. Enter an amount in the Amount field. The bottom section of the Receive Payment window displays any other dependants on the account. The account payment is evenly distributed over each balance or you can manually distribute the payment among the account members.
6. Before processing the payment, select the *Print Payment Receipt* check box.
7. Select *OK* to process the payment. A window appears asking whether you are ready to apply the payment. Select *Yes*.

EagleSoft Online User's Guide

It is recommended that you become familiar with how to run certain parts of the EagleSoft program before beginning your assignments. You will want to review the *Online User's Guide* for these topics:

- New Patient Setup
- OnSchedule Setup
- Scheduling Appointments
- Account Ledger
- Account Window

Online User's Guide – Once you have started EagleSoft, select *Help* above the toolbar, and then select *User's Guide*. To find specific information, select the *Index* tab. You will then be able to enter a keyword to find the appropriate section(s) in the Help box. Double-click the sub-entry (if present) that best describes the subject with which you need help. The requested Help Topic window will appear and may be printed for easy reference.

Access Patterson EagleSoft's online knowledge base by going to *Online → FAQ*. Search FAQ to find the answers to some of the most common questions. The most commonly requested topics have been reprinted for your convenience. You may also visit this information online at http://bit.ly/ES_FAQ.

Reviewing Account Ledger

The Account Ledger section shows all transactions that have been posted to any member in the selected account. The most recent transactions are listed at the top, and the default OnSchedule colors are listed near the bottom. These colors can be changed by going to *File → Preferences → Accounting → Ledger Colors* button.

- All debit transactions (transactions that increase the patient's balance) and notes are displayed in black (for example, patient services are in black).
- All transactions with outstanding insurance claims appear in blue.
- All credit transactions (transactions that decrease the patient's balance) are displayed in red (for example, patient's payment appears in red).
- Deleted transactions and adjustments are in green. A deletion adjustment refers to the offsetting adjustment that is created by deleting an original transaction. For example:
  Deleting a $100 service, which is a debit amount, creates a $100 Delete Adjustment, which is a credit amount.
  Deleting a $50 payment, which is a credit amount, creates a $50 Delete Adjustment, which is a debit amount to offset the original transaction.

A running balance is kept and displayed. Following is a listing of the various types of Debit Transactions:
- Completed service
- Debit adjustment
- Billing charge
- Finance charge
- Returned check

The following listing encompasses the various types of Credit Transactions:
- Account payments
- Insurance payments
- Payment plan payments
- Credit adjustment
- Write off of the account

In addition to debit and credit transactions, the account history also displays the following types of account notes:
- Account note
- Modified transactions
- Deleted transactions
- Submitted insurance notes
- Payment plans
- Letters, recalls, and statements

Accepting an Account Payment or Payment on a Payment Plan

1. From the Account window, choose *Acct Payment*. The Account Payment window is displayed. You can also access this by right-clicking in the Patient window in the Account window.
2. If the patient has a payment plan, click the *Payment Plan* radio button.
3. Type in the payment information. Reminder: Payments are assigned to the oldest patient balance first, unless specified otherwise.
4. Choose *OK* to record the payment and return to the Account window.

New Patient Setup

1. From the Lists menu, choose *Practice Management Lists* and then *Person* or click *Person* on the toolbar
   -or
2. In Practice Management or Clinical modes, select *Person* from the Lists menu. The Person List window is displayed.
3. To add a new patient, choose *New*. The New Person window is displayed.

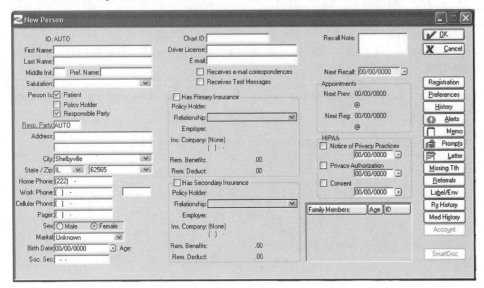

4. Enter the ID. The ID can include numbers or letters up to five characters. If you have chosen auto numbering, the ID is automatically entered for you after you save the information. Once the ID is saved, it cannot be changed without deleting the patient.
5. Enter the name of the patient and type or select the salutation. The salutation is used on letters generated in EagleSoft.
6. Enter the patient's preferred name and middle initial.
7. Indicate whether this person is a Responsible Party, Policy Holder, or Patient by checking the appropriate boxes. If the person is only a policy holder for the account and not a patient, this person must still be set up within EagleSoft; just designate the person as a policy holder only. The same holds true for a person acting as a responsible party. An example might be a parent who is not a patient at your practice, but has a child who is a patient at your practice. In this situation, add the parent to your database and designate the parent as a responsible party for the patient.
8. If the patient is not a responsible party, then type the responsible party's ID. (Press the *F2* key to choose or create a responsible party.) The responsible party's name is displayed.
9. Type or select the patient's other biographical information, such as the Social Security number and birth date.
10. Enter a Chart ID record for additional sorting and filtering options.
11. Enter the patient's Driver's License number.
12. Type or select the *Recall Note, Next Recall* date, and *Next Prev Appt* (next preventive appointment) date.
    - **Recall Note** is used to identify specific patients. For example, if you type the word *CROWN,* you can later generate a report in Money Finder of all patients with the *CROWN* recall note.
    - **Next Prev Appointment** date is the manually entered date for the next preventive appointment (if you are not using OnSchedule) or the next preventive appointment date with an appointment type marked to update the next preventive appointment (for OnSchedule users).
    - **Next Regular Appointment** date is the manually entered date for the next regular appointment (if you are not using OnSchedule) or the next regular appointment date with an appointment type marked to update the next regular appointment (for OnSchedule users).
13. Mark the box *Has Primary Insurance,* if applicable.
14. Enter the Policy Holder ID (or press *F2* to select or create a policy holder).
15. Specify the relationship to the insured and the employer providing insurance. Press *F2* to select an existing employer or to create a new one.
16. Verify the Rem. Benefits (Remaining Benefits) and Rem. Deduct (Remaining Deductible), if applicable.
17. If the patient has secondary insurance, choose *Has Secondary Insurance.* You are asked if you would like to assign the person as the secondary policy holder. If someone other than this person is the secondary policy holder, choose *No;* otherwise, choose *Yes.*

18. Type or select the *Recall Note, Next Recall* date, (next preventive appointment). Next Recall date is typically the date in which the patient is due for his/her next prophy appointment. However, if using Multiple Recalls the patient's Default recall type will show. Click on the Recall Type hyperlink to view all Recall Types for the patient.
19. View the patient's next scheduled appointments.
20. Select the checkbox, under HIPAA, to save the date of Notice of Privacy Policy, Privacy Authorization, and Consent.
21. View a list of family members with scheduled appointments. Right-click to open OnSchedule.
22. Add and view Patient photos in Practice Management. In Edit Person, click the *New Patient Photo* button and browse to the photo location. Select the patient photo file and click *OK*.
23. Choose *OK* to save and return to the Person List window.

OnSchedule Setup

Before you begin scheduling appointments, you must first specify some preferences for using OnSchedule in your office. To utilize OnSchedule to its fullest, please take the time to set up the following:

Scheduler Preferences

To set up your preferences for OnSchedule:
1. From the File menu, choose *Preferences* and click *OnSchedule*.
2. See the section on Preferences for more information on setting up OnSchedule preferences.

Provider Hours

To set up provider hours:
1. From the Practice Management Lists menu, select *Provider/Staff*.
2. From the Providers/Staff List box, highlight the provider to whom you assign hours and click *Edit*.
3. From the Edit Provider/Staff window, click *Hours*. The Provider Hours window is displayed. Adjust the hours as necessary, and click *OK*.
4. The color used in OnSchedule to identify this provider is shown in the Provider Color on Schedule box.
5. To change the color for the provider, click *Change Color*. The Colors window opens. Click on the new color of your choice, and then click *OK*. The new color appears in the Provider Color on Schedule box.
   Note: EagleSoft does not recommend the use of darker colors for the providers.
6. Modify the Start, Close, and Lunch times for the provider. If the provider does not work on a day the practice is open, uncheck the box next to the name of the day, removing the checkmark next to *Open*.
7. If the provider is unavailable for lunch times, be sure the box next to *Take Lunch* is checked and that the lunch times are accurate for this provider.
8. Complete the steps above for each of the days the provider is/is not available.

1 Dentistry as a Business

Although you currently may not work in a dental business office, you must recognize that the administrative professional's role in a dental office of the twenty-first century is one that will continue to change and be challenging. You will certainly need to have a familiarity with a dental business office, and understand the role of a dental business office. Review Chapter 1 in the textbook, and then progress through this workbook chapter to ensure that you are familiar with the material in the textbook and are ready to function in a dental business office.

LEARNING OUTCOMES

On completion of text and workbook chapters, the student should be able to do the following:
- Define key terms.
- Explain the dual role of dentistry as a business and a healthcare service.
- Describe the importance of patient service.
- Define *organizational culture*.
- Describe common organizational cultures that could exist in a dental practice.
- Define communication.
- Differentiate between leadership and management.
- Identify common leadership traits.
- Describe management responsibilities.
- List characteristics necessary for establishing relationships.

SHORT-ANSWER OR FILL-IN QUESTIONS

1. Complete the blank spaces in the diagram shown below.

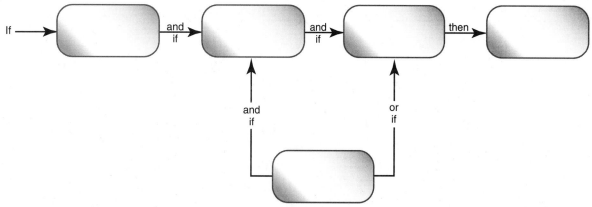

The service concept.

2. Explain in two or more sentences the importance of the service concept to the practice of dentistry. What would happen in the practice if the patient is not satisfied with the service?

_____

_____

_____

_____

3. Identify 10 activities that can promote service.

1. _____

2. _____

3. _____

4. _____

5. _____

6. _____

7. _____

8. _____

9. _____

10. _____

4. List in column A some of the tasks or activities that are common to a business, such as selling a product. Then in Column B list some of the tasks or activities that are common to the practice of dentistry. What are the similarities?

Column A   **Column B**

_____   _____

_____   _____

_____   _____

_____   _____

_____   _____

_____   _____

_____   _____

_____   _____

_____   _____

5. How do the activities in Question 4, Column A, differ from those in Column B? What are the similarities? What are the differences? Can you now explain why dentistry is a business?

_____

_____

_____

_____

_____

6. From your response to Question 5, what can you conclude about the interrelationship between dentistry and business?

_____

_____

7. Differentiate between *management* and *leadership*.

_____

_____

_____

_____

_____

8. What makes an effective leader? After answering this question, determine whether you could be an effective leader. If you answer *no*, identify why not and determine what it would take for you to become an effective leader.

_____

_____

_____

_____

_____

9. Define *organizational culture*.

_____

_____

_____

10. List and describe six types of organizational culture.

1. _____

_____

2. _____

_____

3. _____

_____

4. _____

_____

5. _____

_____

6. _____

_____

Choose three and explain how these cultures function.

1. _____

_____

2. _____

_____

3. _____

_____

11. Why is it important to understand the type of organizational culture that exists in a practice where you may be employed?

_____

_____

MULTIPLE-CHOICE QUESTIONS

12. What term can best describe how to retain patients in a dental practice?
    a. Profit margin
    b. Types of dental materials
    c. Communication
    d. Staffing practices

13. The organizational culture style where people become bogged down with how things are done, not with what is achieved is known as _____ culture.
    a. leadership
    b. blame
    c. power
    d. process

14. Which of the following tasks would *not* indicate that a dentist employer is taking the actions to empower the staff:
    a. Limit employees' access to information that will help them increase their productivity and effectiveness.
    b. Allow staff members to take on more responsibility.
    c. Assign all legal tasks delegated in a given state.
    d. Allow staff members to have a voice in decision making.

15. Which of these is *not* a characteristic that leads to successful risk-taking?
    a. Trusting in one's own abilities
    b. Being open-minded
    c. Overcoming the fear of mistakes
    d. Being dependent on others

16. A good listener _____.
    a. hears the facts as well as the feelings behind the facts
    b. listens strongly with the ears only
    c. avoids becoming involved with the other person
    d. maintains a sense of an advisory capacity

1. Discuss situations in a dental office that are more effective when performed as a team. Why is the team so important in these situations?

2. Think back on work or school relationships that you have had over the years. Reflect on the various personal characteristics that have developed during this experience, and determine what made the good relationships effective and how the negative relationships could have been improved to become more positive.

3. Consider offices that you have visited and determine whether there is effective leadership in the office. How does the leader disseminate a practice vision to the staff?

4. Reflect on past job situations, and determine how the various personal characteristics of an office manager affected how you developed a positive or negative relationship with the staff.

2 Dental Team Management

This chapter deals with dental team management—the manner in which the practice is operated and how the dental staff members work together to enable the practice to grow. To function smoothly, a set of goals and objectives must be in place, and it is vital that the dentist in a healthcare practice seek input from the staff when establishing these objectives. Review the chapter, and then complete the questions in this workbook to ensure that you have a thorough understanding of the concepts and practices used in dental team management.

LEARNING OUTCOMES

On completion of the text and workbook chapters, the student should be able to do the following:
- Define key terms.
- Determine goals and objectives for a dental practice.
- Explain *business etiquette*.
- List the duties of an administrative assistant.
- Identify the five *Rs* of good management.
- Identify the functions of an administrative assistant.
- Identify the characteristics of an effective administrative assistant.
- Manage interpersonal communications of the staff and dentist.
- Explain *employee empowerment*.
- Discuss the procedures for conducting a staff meeting.
- Explain the importance of hiring a skilled administrative assistant.
- Define *time management*.
- Describe how to manage time efficiently.
- Explain the purpose of an office procedural manual.
- Identify components of an office procedural manual.
- Describe recruitment and hiring practices.
- Describe the contents of a personnel policy in an office procedural manual.
- Explain the use of pre-employment testing.
- Describe new employee orientation.
- Manage staff conflict.

SHORT-ANSWER OR FILL-IN QUESTIONS

1. What three steps should a dentist do before opening a dental practice?

    1. _____

    2. _____

    3. _____

2. Define *business etiquette*, and explain why it impacts the success of a dental practice.

    _____

    _____

    _____

    _____

3. List 10 suggestions for implementing good business etiquette in the dental practice.

1. _____

2. _____

3. _____

4. _____

5. _____

6. _____

7. _____

8. _____

9. _____

10. _____

4. List and define the five *R*s of management.

1. _____

_____

2. _____

_____

3. _____

_____

4. _____

_____

5. _____

_____

5. In the circular diagram below, insert the basic functions of an administrative assistant (a), and explain why a circular pattern best describes these functions (b).

a.

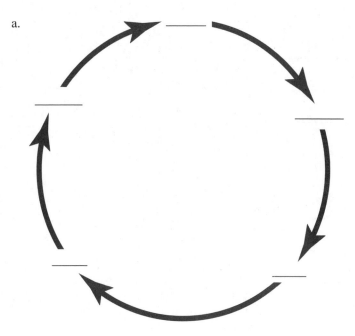

Functions of an administrative assistant.

b. _____

_____

6. List and describe four basic skills a successful administrative assistant should possess. Which of these skills do you possess? If you do not have one of these skills, how could you develop it?

1. _____

_____

2. _____

_____

3. _____

_____

4. _____

_____

7. List 10 attributes that a caring, ethical administrative assistant should possess.

1. _____

2. _____

3. _____

4. _____

5. _____

6. _____

7. _____

8. _____

9. _____

10. _____

8. Informal channels of communication in a dental office can be referred to as _____ communication.

9. Daily, scheduled staff meetings before seeing patients each day is a _____ type of meeting.

10. A staff meeting should provide an opportunity to define and review the goals for the practice and maintain an _____ channel of communication.

11. When investigating a complaint, an administrative assistant should do the following:

1. _____

2. _____

3. _____

12. Why is time management so important to the success of an administrative assistant in a dental practice?

_____

_____

_____

13. List six time wasters in Column A and the solutions that can prevent each of them in Column B.

Column A

1. _____

2. _____

3. _____

4. _____

5. _____

6. _____

Column B

_____

_____

_____

_____

_____

_____

MULTIPLE-CHOICE QUESTIONS

14. It is 8:00 AM on Tuesday in your office, and the following tasks need to be accomplished today. Choose the order with which they most likely would be performed using the concepts of time management.
    1. Schedule a flight for the doctor to go to a technical meeting next Friday.
    2. Send a fax to an oral surgeon with information about a patient who is to have oral surgery at 4:00 PM today.
    3. Call a patient to check on his or her progress after undergoing extensive rehabilitative treatment yesterday.
    4. Call a patient to fill a cancellation for 10:00 AM today.
       a. 2, 4, 3, 1
       b. 3, 1, 2, 4
       c. 4, 1, 2, 3
       d. 4, 2, 3, 1

15. Which of the following would *not* be a part of a job analysis?
    a. Observe the employee performing the job.
    b. List the tasks that make up the job.
    c. Determine the skills and personality characteristics needed for the job.
    d. Determine the age and education needed for the job.

16. The form completed by candidates is Immigration and Naturalization Service (INS) Form I-9 (Employment Eligibility Verification form). The form used by an employer to prove an applicant's legal status, is a/an:
    a. W-2
    b. I-9
    c. I-4
    d. W-4

17. A new clerical staff person is working in the business office and lays the health questionnaire of another patient on the counter in the view of a patient who is being dismissed. What should the administrative assistant do?
    a. Grab it out of the view of the patient and immediately inform the clerical person in front of the staff never to lay such forms within the view of another person.
    b. Ignore that the form is there and assume that the patient being dismissed did not see it.
    c. Retrieve the form and talk to the clerical person privately about confidentiality and the risk of placing such a record in the view of another person.
    d. Retrieve the form and bring the issue up in the next monthly staff meeting.

18. Mutual trust or emotional relationship that exists among the office staff members is referred to as which of the following?
    a. Respect
    b. Rapport
    c. Rationale
    d. Recognition

19. Which of the following questions should be avoided during a personal job interview?
    a. Tell me about your previous work experience.
    b. Tell me about your marriage.
    c. What have your previous educational experiences been?
    d. What are your career goals?

20. Which of the following questions should be avoided during a job interview?
    a. What was your absentee record at your prior place of employment?
    b. Would you be able to work in a satellite office 10 miles from this location?
    c. Are you available to work overtime?
    d. Which religious holidays do you practice?

CRITICAL THINKING ACTIVITIES

1. Describe how you would handle the following conflict situations:
    a. Dr. Lake reprimands you for not making a telephone that call he requested you to make. What would you do?

    b. During a lunch break, a chair-side or clinical assistant criticizes another assistant for wearing facial piercings, which is a violation of the office procedural manual for clinical assistants. You are the administrative assistant and are part of the lunch group. What would be your response?

    c. You are the administrative assistant in an office where the office hours for the staff are 8:15 AM to 5:00 PM. An assistant is chronically late, arriving 15 to 20 minutes after the assigned time each day. This employee performs her clinical tasks well and has a good rapport with the patients. She states she must always leave by 5:00 PM and seldom is late leaving for lunch. Friction is occurring among the staff. The dentist does not seem to be concerned. Is this really a problem? What are the issues involved? Can there be a resolution? What action should be taken, and who should take the action?

d. A new clerical assistant, Tina, in the business office places a health questionnaire from a new patient on the counter where patients who are being dismissed normally stand to make appointments. One of the senior business assistants, Wanda, tells her in a stern voice that can be heard by others that she should not have done that. Tina is embarrassed and quickly grabs the form and takes it away. How could this incident have been handled in a better manner?

e. You have just been assigned the new position of administrative assistant in the dental office where you are employed. There has never been an office procedural manual. The doctor asks you to provide an outline for such a manual and to research the existence of samples of such manuals from any sources available, if possible. Put together the materials you are able to find in your area, and provide a sample of an outline for an office procedural manual that could be used in the office in which you are or might be employed.

3 Patient Management

People are an essential part of the dental practice. The most important person in a dental practice is the patient. Therefore it is vital that the administrative assistant develop an understanding of patient management. The dental professional is faced with a variety of personalities, backgrounds, and patients with special needs. No single method serves all people when it comes to communication. However, while communicating with patients, it is important to recognize each patient as an individual with specific needs and to determine how to be sensitive to those needs. Remember that dentistry is a "helping" profession. Not only must every effort be made to alleviate patients' discomfort, but patients must be taught to help themselves. After reviewing the chapter in the textbook, complete the questions in this workbook chapter to ensure that you have a basic understanding of how to manage the needs of a variety of patients. In addition, you should be able to create communication tools to promote patient understanding and to market the practice.

LEARNING OUTCOMES

On completion of text and workbook chapters, the student should be able to do the following:
- Define key terms.
- Understand patient needs.
- Explain the special needs of patients.
- Identify barriers to communication.
- Recognize nonverbal cues.
- Manage interpersonal communication in the reception area.
- Design an office policy statement.
- Explain marketing techniques in dentistry.
- Describe external and internal marketing.
- Understand patient rights.

SHORT-ANSWER OR FILL-IN QUESTIONS

1. In the graphic below, an illustration of Maslow's hierarchy of needs, insert the names of the various levels.

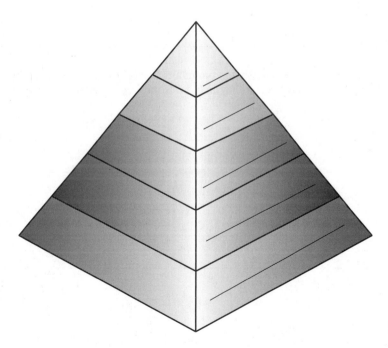

Maslow's hierarchy of needs.

2. Explain two basic types of marketing procedures that could be used in a dental practice.

1. _____

_____

_____

2. _____

_____

_____

3. List five ideas that could be implemented in a dental practice to increase marketing for existing patients.

1. _____

2. _____

3. _____

4. _____

5. _____

4. Which five activities could attract new patients?

1. _____

2. _____

3. _____

4. _____

5. _____

5. Describe five different situations that would illustrate barriers to communication. These examples may be patient-oriented situations that occur in a typical dental practice, or they may be from life experiences outside the dental office.

1. _____

2. _____

3. _____

4. _____

5. _____

6. During your daily activities, become aware of nonverbal cues given to you. What types of facial expressions, hand movements, and torso movements do you notice? Do they affect your behavior?

_____

_____

_____

7. List 10 rights that a person has as a patient in the dental practice.

1. _____

2. _____

3. _____

4. _____

5. _____

6. _____

7. _____

8. _____

9. _____

10. _____

8. What is the purpose of an office policy?

_____

_____

9. List eight items that might be included in an office policy.

1. _____

2. _____

3. _____

4. _____

5. _____

6. _____

7. _____

8. _____

10. Explain how a newsletter can become a valuable marketing tool.

_____

_____

_____

MULTIPLE-CHOICE QUESTIONS

11. When a person has reached the _____ level on Maslow's hierarchy of needs, he or she is said to have sufficiently satisfied the basic needs and is motivated to help others achieve their goals by teaching them lessons learned in the earlier stages. Some people never reach this level because they have not aspired to its recognition.
    a. physiological
    b. self-actualization
    c. social
    d. ego

12. Which of the following is *not* a patient's right?
    a. To be treated with adequate, appropriate, compassionate care at all times and under all circumstances
    b. To be treated without discrimination based on race, religion, color, national origin, gender, age, handicap, marital status, sexual preference, or source of payment
    c. To be informed of aspects of treatment
    d. To be informed of comparison community fees for the recommended service

13. The patient has the right to each of the following *except*:
    a. To be able to review the financial and clinical records
    b. To receive the original copies of all reports and radiographs or other documents on request
    c. To be treated as a partner in the care and decision making related to treatment planning
    d. To obtain a thorough evaluation of his or her needs

14. A patient has the right to _____ treatment but must be informed of the _____ of that refusal.

    The patient must then _____ a refusal for treatment form or document and it is then recorded in the

    _____.
    a. refuse, medical or dental consequences, sign, clinical record
    b. refuse, financial cost, sign, financial record
    c. accept, medical or dental consequences, pay for, clinical record
    d. accept, financial cost, sign, financial record

15. Which of the following is a common indication of abuse in a child?
    a. Smiling
    b. Stunted growth
    c. Dental caries
    d. Bruises of varying colors on exposed areas of the body

16. Which of the following is *not* acceptable protocol for professional etiquette in the dental office?
    a. Using correct grammar
    b. Standing as close as possible to a person engaged in conversation with another person
    c. Eating or drinking in the staff lounge
    d. Excusing yourself to answer the telephone

17. An office policy differs from an office procedural manual in which of the following ways?
    a. It is designed for patients and informs them of the protocols of the office and its staff.
    b. It is designed for staff use and includes office rules and regulations.
    c. It is a statement of financial management and insurance policies.
    d. It is a listing of all staff members and contact information.

18

18. A form of therapy that when applied to dentistry encourages listening to patients to learn about their feelings, desires, and priorities is referred to as which of the following?
    a. Maslow's hierarchy of needs
    b. Client-centered therapy
    c. Self-actualized therapy
    d. Interactive therapy

19. Newsletters may be considered for all of the following reasons *except*:
    a. They represent an internal market that is sent to current patients.
    b. Newsletters are part of the external market because they are sent to the nearby community and addressed to the resident at the given address.
    c. Newsletters contribute to the education of the public.
    d. They are the least expensive form of advertising.

20. Which of the following is *not* true regarding the observation of abuse in a patient?
    a. The dentist has an obligation to examine the patient thoroughly.
    b. The dentist needs to ask reasonable questions about existing conditions and to document the injuries on the dental record.
    c. Reports of suspected abuse should be made to the state or county social services office.
    d. In most states failure to report suspected abuse is a felony.

CRITICAL THINKING ACTIVITIES

1. Consider Maslow's hierarchy and decide first where you are on the hierarchy and why you think this is true. Then decide what it will take in your life to move to the next higher level. Do you want to move to the next level? Are you satisfied to be at the level you are now?

2. If a clinical facility is available, observe nonverbal behavior. Silently stand out of sight of a patient, dentist or dental student, and a dental auxiliary. Observe as many forms of nonverbal communication as possible. Did the participants pick up these clues? If so, what was the reaction?

3. How can you become a practice ambassador for your employer?

4 Legal and Ethical Issues in the Dental Business Office

As a dental practice administrative assistant, you will be faced with issues involving the legal requirements and standards of care, voluntary and involuntary, in the delivery of dental treatment each day. Each person in a dental practice must be acutely aware of the dental law within his or her state. Further, each person should understand the profession's principles of ethics, voluntary standards, and how these apply to the practice. These legal and voluntary requirements are in place to protect society and patients in the dental practice. Thus to be certain that you understand the basics of the legal and ethical issues in the dental practice, review the textbook chapter and then complete this workbook chapter.

LEARNING OUTCOMES

On completion of text and workbook chapters, the student should be able to do the following:
- Define key terms.
- Explain the impact of ethics and law on the dental business office.
- Differentiate between the various types of law that affect the practice of dentistry.
- Explain various types of consent.
- Describe situations in the dental business office that would lead to potential litigation.
- Describe the code of ethics of professional dental organizations.
- Identify 12 steps in making ethical decisions.

SHORT-ANSWER OR FILL-IN QUESTIONS

1. The three forms of consent that exist in the delivery of dental care are _____ _____, _____ _____, and _____ _____.

2. Which four questions should be asked to determine an unintentional tort of negligence in dental care?

    1. _____

    2. _____

    3. _____

    4. _____

3. Identify 10 steps that should be followed in the making of ethical decisions.

    1. _____

    2. _____

    3. _____

    4. _____

    5. _____

    6. _____

7. _____

8. _____

9. _____

10. _____

4. Identify 10 implied duties that a dentist owes a patient.

 1. _____

 2. _____

 3. _____

 4. _____

 5. _____

 6. _____

 7. _____

 8. _____

 9. _____

 10. _____

5. Explain informed consent.

_____

_____

_____

_____

6. Explain the function of a state dental practice act and its impact on a consumer.

_____

_____

7. List 10 acts that could lead to potential negligence.

 1. _____

 2. _____

 3. _____

 4. _____

5. _____

6. _____

7. _____

8. _____

9. _____

10. _____

8. Define the elements of informed consent.

_____

_____

_____

_____

9. Define each of the following acronyms:

ADA _____

ADAA _____

ADHA _____

DANB _____

AADOM _____

MATCHING EXERCISE

10. Match the following terms in Column A with the correct definitions in Column B.

Column A	**Column B**
_____ Dental Practice Act	a. Immunity for acts performed by a person who renders care in an emergency situation
_____ Civil law	b. Central repository to collect and release information on professional competence and conduct
_____ Criminal law	c. The person or party that institutes the suit in court
_____ Misdemeanor	d. Relates to duties between persons or between citizens and their government
_____ Felony	e. Wrongs committed against the public as a whole
_____ Intentional	f. Treatment that a reasonable person would perform in similar circumstances
_____ Standard of care	g. A less serious crime, which is punishable by a fine or imprisonment for less than a year
_____ Negligence	h. Legal requirements necessary to practice developed through legislative action within the state

Chapter **4** **Legal and Ethical Issues in the Dental Business Office**

_____	Malpractice	i.	The performance of an act that a reasonably careful person under similar circumstances would not do or, conversely, would do
_____	Litigation	j.	More serious crime, which is punishable by imprisonment for more than a year
_____	Lawsuit	k.	Negligence by professionals but can mean, in a broader sense, any wrongdoing by professionals
_____	Plaintiff	l.	The process of a lawsuit
_____	Ethics	m.	Membership in a professional organization
_____	Expert witness	n.	Person being accused of a wrongdoing
_____	Fact witness	o.	When placed under oath, must provide only firsthand knowledge, not hearsay
_____	Defendant	p.	Communication of false information about a person to a third party that results in injury to that person's reputation
_____	Good Samaritan Law	q.	Differentiation between right and wrong
_____	National Practitioner Data Bank	r.	A cost-containment system of managing health benefits
_____	Fraud	s.	Unexcused harmful or offensive physical contact that is intentionally performed
_____	Abandonment	t.	Transferring information to an insurance company about a patient without the patient's consent
_____	Defamation of character	u.	Severance of a professional relationship with a patient who is still in need of dental care and attention without giving adequate notice to the patient
_____	Invasion of privacy	v.	Deception deliberately practiced to secure unfair or unlawful gain
_____	Assault and battery	w.	When testifying, must explain what happened based on the patient's record and offer an opinion as to whether the dental care, as administered, met acceptable standards
_____	Voluntary action	x.	Legal action in a court
_____	Managed care	y.	Planned to commit a wrongful act

MULTIPLE-CHOICE QUESTIONS

11. An assistant is hired in the practice as a clinical dental assistant. The doctor indicates that this person is to place an intracoronal provisional restoration. The person knows how to perform the task but does not yet have the registered dental assistant, or RDA, credential required to perform the specific intraoral task in this state. She asks you, as the administrative assistant, what she should do. You should respond by suggesting that she do what?
    a. She should do what the doctor told her to do.
    b. She should perform the task now but later tell the doctor that she does not have the appropriate credential.
    c. She should inform the doctor that she does not have the appropriate credential to perform this task at this time.
    d. She should perform the task with the self-assurance that she will soon have her credential.

12. Which of the following actions are common negligent acts in a dental office?
    a. Mistaken identity
    b. Defects in equipment
    c. Failure to communicate
    d. Disease transmission
    e. All of the above

13. The Good Samaritan Law provides incentives for healthcare providers to provide medical assistance to the injured without the fear of potential litigation *except* which of the following?
    a. Protection for a negligent healthcare provider who is being compensated for services
    b. Immunity for acts performed by a person who renders care in an emergency situation
    c. When the provider is solely interested in providing care in a safe manner, with no intent to do bodily harm

14. An insurance company requests verification of a patient's birth date and complete name. A copy of the patient's entire record is sent to the company, including a health history that indicates evidence of human immunodeficiency virus (HIV). This action may be considered _____.
    a. fraud
    b. violation of confidentiality
    c. assault and battery
    d. defamation of character

15. The responsibility to be ever mindful of the changes in the laws and societal ethics requires constant _____ on the part of the dental professional.
    a. fear
    b. vigilance
    c. observation
    d. change

CRITICAL THINKING ACTIVITIES

1. A patient is seen in the office where you are employed. The doctor recommends a treatment plan and offers alternative treatment that includes identification of the risks involved. The patient declines to have any of the treatment completed. This discussion is not recorded in the record. Then 5 years later the doctor receives notice that she is involved in litigation for this patient. The patient claims that he never knew the consequences of his neglect. What is the doctor's defense? What should have been done at the conclusion of the consultation to avoid such action?

2. You are to testify in a malpractice case regarding the insertion of an implant that has been made against your dentist employer. At the time of the treatment, you were the administrative assistant. Another assistant, Mary Tombs, CDA (certified dental assistant), was the clinical assistant. Mary observed the treatment, and you were asked to record the treatment on the patient's clinical record. Dr. Fredrik Voltema, professor of prosthetic dentistry at the University of Tremont School of Dentistry, has also been asked to testify in this case. Which of the following statements is/are true? Explain your choice of answers.
    a. Mary Tombs is an expert witness because she assisted the dentist in the insertion of the implant.
    b. Dr. Fredrik Voltema is a professor of dentistry in prosthetics and is an expert witness.
    c. The administrative assistant is a fact witness.

Chapter **4** **Legal and Ethical Issues in the Dental Business Office**

1. Complete an Internet search at www.danb.org, and determine the dental assisting job titles and the educational and licensure requirements, if any, for a dental assistant for your current state of residence and two other states where you might consider employment.

2. Visit www.ada.org/prof/prac/law/code/ on the Internet, and identify the three main components of the American Dental Association Principles of Ethics and Code of Professional Conduct. Then select *The Public* tab, from which you can choose two or more areas or topics to browse. Determine how these public areas would affect dental professional education. Why is this web site so important for the dental professional? What did you learn while visiting this site? How could this web site be used for the dental business office administrative assistant?

5 | Technology in the Business Office

The modern dental business office contains a multitude of office technologies. Today's dental administrative assistant must be familiar with the technology and accustomed to using each facet of it so that the staff can be productive and the dentist will remain on the cutting edge. Technology in the office is the application of computers and associated electronic equipment to prepare and distribute information. Review the textbook chapter, and become familiar with the application of the computer to the dental practice. Then complete the following questions as they relate to this chapter.

LEARNING OUTCOMES

On completion of the text and workbook chapters, the student should be able to do the following:
- Define key terms.
- Differentiate between a manual office and an office using the latest technology.
- List types of electronic office equipment used in technology.
- Describe the elements of information systems.
- Explain the four operations of a computer.
- Explain how technology can be used to increase profitability.
- Describe the application of technology to a dental practice.
- Explain the purpose of a feasibility study.
- Explain the difference between general and specific task software.
- Discuss dental software, word processing, electronic spreadsheet, database, graphics, and Internet software.
- List the guidelines to follow when selecting software.
- Explain why implementing a change to a computer system is important to all staff members.

SHORT-ANSWER OR FILL-IN QUESTIONS

1. List the five elements that constitute an information system.

    1. _____

    2. _____

    3. _____

    4. _____

    5. _____

2. List and describe the four general operations of a computer that are known as the *information processing cycle*.

    1. _____

    2. _____

    3. _____

    4. _____

3. The mouse to the computer in the business office is broken and needs to be replaced. Discuss some options that could be featured in a replacement mouse.

_____

_____

_____

_____

4. List 10 applications of computer technology in the dental office.

   1. _____

   2. _____

   3. _____

   4. _____

   5. _____

   6. _____

   7. _____

   8. _____

   9. _____

  10. _____

5. Discuss five or six guidelines that should be used in making the right software selection for a dental practice.

   1. _____

     _____

   2. _____

     _____

   3. _____

     _____

   4. _____

     _____

5. _____

_____

6. _____

_____

MATCHING EXERCISE

6. Match the term in Column A with the definition in Column B.

Column A	Column B
_____ Hardware	a. Carried by members of the office staff, allows them to be signaled when needed
_____ Computer	b. Worldwide collection of networks that connects millions of businesses and individuals
_____ Voicemail	c. A series of instructions that tells a computer what to do and how to do it
_____ Pager	d. Physical equipment
_____ Fax machine	e. A type of software enabling one to produce written communication
_____ Digital camera	f. Input text or graphical data directly into computer storage
_____ Cosmetic imager	g. Device that electronically accepts, processes, provides output, and stores data
_____ Scanner	h. Facts or figures that the information system needs to produce accurate and timely information
_____ Word processor	i. Allows both incoming and outgoing telephone messages to be recorded and processed
_____ Data	j. Allow images to become part of the patient record
_____ Byte	k. Send and receive documents or other graphical images over the telephone systems or the Internet
_____ Internet	l. Portable miniature mobile storage device that can fit on key chain
_____ Shredder	m. Displays proposed changes that will result from specific treatment
_____ Software	n. A device that destroys documents to guard against identity theft and protect confidentiality
_____ Flash (jump) drive	o. Roughly equivalent to one character of text

MULTIPLE-CHOICE QUESTIONS

7. Computer literacy involves having current knowledge and understanding of which of the following?
   a. Computer programming
   b. Computers and their uses
   c. Computer repair
   d. All of the above

8. _____ is/are a collection of unprocessed items that can include text, numbers, images, audio, and video.
   a. Information
   b. Instructions
   c. Programs
   d. Data

9. _____ controls the resources on a network.
   a. Workstation
   b. Server
   c. Client
   d. Tower

10. A gigabyte (GB) is approximately how many numbers of bytes?
    a. One thousand
    b. One million
    c. One billion
    d. One trillion

11. A patient information screen in dental software will provide which of the following?
    a. All the clinical data about the patient
    b. Only the current clinical data that are incomplete
    c. Comprehensive personal and financial patient information
    d. Only the current balance of the financial record

12. Which would likely be the two most common violations of computer ethics in the dental office?
    a. Software theft and piracy
    b. Hardware theft and piracy
    c. License burning and software theft
    d. Copyright violations and piracy

13. For which of the following systems is the computer used the least in the dental office?
    a. Treatment records
    b. Financial records
    c. Recall
    d. Inventory

14. Which of the following screens would provide information about a patient who has incomplete work and has missed, canceled, or broken appointments?
    a. Treatment plan
    b. Tickler file
    c. Daily appointment
    d. Recall

15. An integrated software system that can graphically demonstrate patient bone loss is available where?
    a. Basic electronic spreadsheet
    b. Periodontal examination and charting system
    c. Basic charting system
    d. Periodontal spreadsheet

16. Which of the following word-processing features enables a person to change the line spacing in a document?
    a. Insert
    b. Delete
    c. Format
    d. Search and replace

17. You wish to locate a word in a document before removing it. Which feature would you use?
    a. Edit and find
    b. Cut and paste
    c. Format and cut
    d. Edit and paste

CRITICAL THINKING ACTIVITIES

1. Think about the offices with which you have had contact in dentistry. Are they paperless? Do you think they soon will become paperless? What areas are difficult to transfer to this concept?

2. If you become employed in an office where the computer appears to be outdated and downtimes are frequent, it may be time to examine the situation with a feasibility study. What are some of the issues that should be considered in such a study? How could you initiate the study?

INTERNET ASSIGNMENT

Many types of software packages are available for use in the modern dental office. Take some time to do an Internet search by entering the phrase *dental software* into a search engine to see what is available on the market. Use an inquiring mind to compare these products, and determine which ones might be worth evaluating for use in a dental practice.

6 Office Design and Equipment Placement

There is nothing more pleasant than to walk into a facility that is beautifully decorated and the reception area exudes warmth. As the administrative assistant, you may have some time to impact the design and efficiency of the reception room and business office in the dental practice where you are employed. For the business office, these responsibilities demand an understanding of the principles of motion economy and the placement of office equipment to create an environment in which a person can work smarter, not harder. Review this chapter in the accompanying textbook, and answer the following questions to ensure your understanding of the content of the chapter.

LEARNING OUTCOMES

On completion of text and workbook chapters, the student should be able to do the following:
- Define key terms.
- Define *ergonomics* as it applies to the dental business office.
- Describe classifications of motion.
- Describe the implementation of time and motion in a dental business office.
- Describe *seasonal affective disorder*.
- Explain the effect of the Americans with Disabilities Act (ADA) on office design.
- Explain a work triangle as it relates to the dental business office.
- Identify criteria for reception room design.
- Identify criteria for business office design.
- Describe factors involved in office design that relate to the ADA.
- Describe the arrangement of common business equipment.

SHORT-ANSWER OR FILL-IN QUESTIONS

1. Define *ergonomics*.

   _____

   _____

2. Describe the concept of time and motion as it applies to a dental business office.

   _____

   _____

3. What ideas might you include in a reception room that would enhance patient comfort?

   _____

   _____

4. List 10 factors that might be considered in designing a business office work environment that would adhere to motion economy, space planning, health issues, and safety.

   1. _____

   _____

   2. _____

   _____

   3. _____

   _____

   4. _____

   _____

   5. _____

   _____

   6. _____

   _____

   7. _____

   _____

   8. _____

   _____

   9. _____

   _____

   10. _____

   _____

5. List five design features that could be included in the office design to provide a barrier-free office.

   1. _____

   2. _____

   3. _____

   4. _____

   5. _____

34

6. Explain five factors that should improve ergonomic body positioning while working in the dental business office.

1. _____

2. _____

3. _____

4. _____

5. _____

MULTIPLE-CHOICE QUESTIONS

7. An ergonomically correct body position for a business assistant when seated at the computer workstation should include all *except* which of the following?
   a. The thighs should be parallel to the floor.
   b. When using the keyboard the arms should be positioned so that the forearms are raised 45 degrees in relation to the keyboard.
   c. The back and neck should be erect.
   d. The upper arms are perpendicular to the floor.

8. To prevent wrist discomfort or possible carpal tunnel syndrome, the business assistant should:
   a. be certain that the keyboard does not tilt.
   b. use an ergonomic mouse or track ball.
   c. use the computer no more than 2 hours in each half day.
   d. wear a wrist brace on the hand used for the mouse.

9. To reduce eyestrain and fatigue when using the computer, the administrative assistant should do all *except* which of the following?
   a. Use good posture.
   b. Periodically look away form the screen for a few minutes.
   c. If using the computer continuously, take a 10- to 15-minute break every hour.
   d. Use an ergonomically designed chair.

10. A direct consequence of seasonal affective disorder (SAD) is:
    a. Winter depression and sleep disorders
    b. Moodiness and weight gain
    c. Summer depression and sleep disorders
    d. State of being alert and awake in the nighttime

11. Class I movement is identified by:
    a. fingers-only movement.
    b. fingers and wrist movement.
    c. fingers, wrist, elbow, and shoulder movement.

12. Which of the following motion classifications should be avoided to improve ergonomic behavior?
    a. Class I
    b. Class II
    c. Class III
    d. Class V

13. Which of the following activities is indicative of a class III movement?
    a. Placing a paper clip on several pages
    b. Answering the telephone
    c. Using a pencil
    d. Turning around and reaching into a cabinet

14. From the list below, select all the true statements that relate to the design of a dental business office and reception room. Place a "T" beside each true statement.

_____ The eye-to-computer screen distance should be 10 to 14 inches.

_____ Doorways should be widened to accommodate wheelchairs and other devices.

_____ Install raised letters; Braille should be placed on elevator controls.

_____ The business office clock should face the reception in full view of patients.

_____ Master controls for the music system, heating, cooling, and lighting also should be located in the reception room.

_____ Lateral or open files require less space than vertical files.

_____ Cupboard space is necessary for storage of paper and supplies.

_____ Telephones should be installed at each workstation and should be made hands free whenever possible.

_____ Desk drawers should not have full suspension.

_____ A small area adjacent to the business office set up for private calls and conversations with patients is convenient and can be used for completion of insurance forms.

_____ The administrative assistant or receptionist should be seated facing the reception room.

_____ The keyboard height level should be approximately 34 inches and the writing level about 29 inches.

_____ An adequate depth for most working areas is 30 inches.

_____ A counter approximately 44 inches high provides a writing area for patients and privacy for the assistant and documents on the desk.

CRITICAL THINKING ACTIVITIES

1. An assistant is hired in your office as a clinical dental assistant. Your office is located in mid-Michigan. This assistant was hired after she had completed an internship through your office as a student during the month of June. During that internship she performed very well and consequently was hired in early September. In late October it was noted that she seemed not to be performing well. You spoke with her about her performance, and she indicated that she liked the work but missed the summer. She tells you that she sometimes wishes she lived in Florida. The doctor tells you that he is thinking of terminating her if she does not improve her attitude. What might be the problem? How could you help this employee? Is there anything that could be done to the physical environment to improve her performance?

2. Using equipment and suggestions from this chapter for office design, develop an office design that might be used for a typical dental practice in your geographic area. Consider the latest electronic equipment, and include suggestions for color and texture of flooring, walls, and lighting. You may want to use graph paper to aid you in placement of office equipment according to size. The size of the business office should be no less that 12 feet × 14 feet. If you wish, you may include exterior windows on one wall. Remember that this will cut down on upper wall shelving or storage.

INTERNET ASSIGNMENT

On the Internet, go to the Americans with Disabilities Act web site (www.ada.gov), and select the link at the top labeled *ADA Design Standards* and then click on the HTML file near the bottom of the screen labeled *ADA Standards for Accessible Design*. From the table of contents, select *Signage* and identify the elements that must be present when posting signs for disabled patients or clients.

7 Working with Dental Office Documents

In reality today's dental office is not paperless, although that may be a dream of every dental professional. The dental office is inundated with many records and forms, all needed as part of the total healthcare and dental business practice. These records are kept so that the office staff can refer to the information later or use it to complete another task. The administrative assistant is required to maintain clinical, financial, employee, state, and federal records. Failure to perform any of these tasks can be a costly experience for the dental practitioner. Take time to thoroughly review the material and forms in this chapter in the textbook. When you are ready, complete the questions in this chapter to ensure your understanding of the contents of this chapter.

LEARNING OUTCOMES

On completion of text and workbook chapters, the student should be able to do the following:
- Define key terms.
- Define *HIPAA*.
- Describe how to implement HIPAA regulations in the dental office record management system.
- Identify the types of records maintained in a dental office.
- Categorize the various types of records.
- Distinguish between *active* and *inactive* records.
- List the components of a clinical record.
- Describe the function of the components of a clinical record.
- Explain the rules for data entry on patient records.
- Explain the use of symbols and abbreviations in clinical records.
- List the components of patient financial records.
- Identify the various types of records required by the Occupational Safety and Health Administration (OSHA) that must be maintained in a dental office.
- Identify the various types of employee records.
- Explain the importance of maintaining accurate records.
- Describe methods of records retention and transfer.

SHORT-ANSWER AND FILL-IN QUESTIONS

1. Define *HIPAA* and explain the responsibility of the administrative assistant to inform a new patient who enters the practice about HIPAA.

_____

_____

_____

_____

_____

_____

2. Describe the difference among vital, important, useful, and nonessential records and give examples of each.

_____

_____

_____

_____

_____

_____

3. List the primary reasons for maintaining accurate clinical records.

_____

_____

_____

_____

_____

4. List 10 items that are vital components of a clinical record.

1. _____

2. _____

3. _____

4. _____

5. _____

6. _____

7. _____

8. _____

9. _____

10. _____

5. List the information that should be included on a chart when treatment has been completed for a patient.

_____

_____

6. Identify five suggestions to follow for efficient and confidential transfer of records from one site to another.

    1. _____

    2. _____

    3. _____

    4. _____

    5. _____

7. a. Using the Universal Numbering System, give the tooth numbers for each of the following permanent teeth:

    Maxillary right first molar   _____

    Mandibular right second premolar   _____

    Maxillary right central incisor   _____

    Maxillary left first premolar   _____

    Mandibular left third molar   _____

   b. Using the Universal Numbering System, give the tooth numbers for each of the following primary teeth:

    Mandibular right canine   _____

    Maxillary right first molar   _____

    Maxillary left central incisor   _____

    Mandibular left second molar   _____

    Mandibular right lateral incisor   _____

8. Indicate the names of the tooth surfaces for each of the following descriptions:

    a. Closest to the midline   _____

    b. Farthest from the midline   _____

    c. Facing the cheeks   _____

    d. Anterior biting edge   _____

    e. Nearest the tongue   _____

9. Provide the clinical abbreviations for the following:

    BID   _____

    TID   _____

Chapter **7 Working with Dental Office Documents**

Br _____

CDA _____

RDH _____

cond _____

evac _____

ext _____

fr _____

imp _____

LLQ _____

OHI _____

Rx _____

Sx _____

TMJ _____

MATCHING

10. From the list in Column A, select the record that best corresponds to the definition in Column B.

Column A	Column B
_____ Medical history form	a. Record that may contain a dental chart, a review of the patient's health history, and general patient information as well as a record of services rendered
_____ Health history update form	b. Used to transfer a patient to another dentist for examination, evaluation, and diagnosis
_____ Registration form	c. Accompanies each case that a dentist sends to a dental laboratory
_____ Medication history form	d. Form that is signed by the patient or guardian of a pediatric patient to grant permission for administration of an anesthetic and other specified procedures
_____ Laboratory prescription or requisition form	e. List of a patient's prescriptions for drugs that could lead to unsafe interactions
_____ Consent form	f. Form that the patient signs to affirm receipt of HIPAA information
_____ Refusal of treatment form	g. Common type of storage for patient records
_____ Consultation and referral report	h. A record of the patient's complete health history
_____ Dental diagnosis and fee estimate form	i. Form that is signed and dated by a patient when the health history and personal information are currently reviewed
_____ File folder or envelope	j. Dentist's findings and treatment plan recommended for the patient
_____ Clinical chart	k. Form that contains general information such as addresses and telephone numbers as well as employment and insurance information
_____ Acknowledgment of receipt and notice of privacy practices	l. Form signed by the patient when he or she does not accept the treatment plan

MULTIPLE-CHOICE QUESTIONS

11. All of the following statements about year aging labels are true *except* which?
    a. Used to identify inactive patient records
    b. Color-coded
    c. Aid in purging records
    d. Used only for active patients

12. Which of the following is *not* a component of a clinical record?
    a. Clinical chart
    b. Health history
    c. Medication history
    d. Ledger card

13. Which of the following is *not true* about a patient history form?
    a. It is reviewed at periodic visits.
    b. It is reviewed for completeness.
    c. It is completed in ink and signed by the patient's legal representative.
    d. Once reviewed and discussed, it is discarded to protect confidentiality.

14. All data entered on a patient's clinical record should be dated, including accurate and complete information, and initialed by the treating dentist and assistant.
    a. True
    b. False

15. How many teeth are present in the primary dentition?
    a. 10
    b. 20
    c. 32
    d. 52

16. How many teeth are present in the permanent dentition?
    a. 10
    b. 20
    c. 32
    d. 52

17. Which of the following tooth numbering systems uses a 1 to 32 numeric system for the permanent dentition?
    a. Universal
    b. Palmer Notation
    c. FDI

18. Which tooth surface is closest to the cheek?
    a. Mesial
    b. Distal
    c. Buccal
    d. Lingual

19. Which of the following is the biting surface of a tooth?
    a. Mesial
    b. Distal
    c. Buccal
    d. Occlusal

20. Dr. Lake asks you to send a case to Parker Dental Laboratory. Complete a laboratory requisition that you obtain from an employer or instructor. Include information from below that was taken from the clinical chart:

John W. Holmes, a male patient, age 36, is to have a porcelain-fused-to-metal (PFM), white high noble crown on the mandibular right first molar. The shade is Vita Lumin C-3. Special instructions should include the following:

- Create a broad contact on the BL and on the occlusal cervical to prevent food impaction.
- No metal band on the B surface and a 1-mm metal collar on the L surface.
- The final cementation appointment is scheduled for 2 weeks from today's date.
- Dr. Lake's license number is 7376, and the office address is 611 Main Street SE, Grand Rapids, MI 49502. The office telephone number is 616-101-9575.

WARD | a dti company

1068 Charles H. Orndorf Drive · Brighton, MI · 48116 · P 810 534 9273 · F 810 534 9278

Crown and Bridge Rx

RX DATE _____

CASE # _____

DATE WANTED	TIME

DOCTOR INFORMATION
Name _____
Address _____
_____
Telephone _____

PATIENT INFORMATION
Name _____
Sex _____ Age _____
○ Diagnostic wax up ○ Pearltemps™ (provisionals)
○ Call me (before proceeding with case)
_____
Rx _____
_____
_____
_____
_____
_____
_____
_____
_____

HAVE YOU INCLUDED THE FOLLOWING?
○ Impression
○ Bite
○ Opposing
○ Shade
○ Pre-op model
○ Photos
○ Model of temps
○ Bite stick
○ Face bow

PLEASE SEND
○ Prescription forms
○ Plastic bags
○ Case boxes

RETURN FOR
○ Die Trim
○ Metal try-in
○ Finish
○ Evaluation
○ Wax check
○ Bisque bake try-in

IF INSUFFICIENT ROOM
○ Reduce and mark
○ Metal occlusion
○ Reduction coping
○ Please call

IF CASE WILL NOT DRAW
○ Make reduction copings
○ Please call

○ Surgical Stent

SHADE _____ STUMP _____

AMOUNT OF TRANSLUCENCY
○ Light   ○ Medium   ○ Heavy

VALUE
○ Bright   ○ Medium   ○ Low

MIDLINE SHIFT
R _____ MM   L _____ MM
_____ MM
Length of centrals from cervical margin
○ Close Diastema

CIRCLE TEETH NUMBERS
1 2 3 4 5 6 7 8 9 10 11 12 13 14 15 16
32 31 30 29 28 27 26 25 24 23 22 21 20 19 18 17

METAL
○ High noble   ○ Noble

OCCLUSION
○ Metal   ○ Porcelain

LATERAL EXCURSION
○ Cuspid guidance   ○ Group function

LABIAL MARGIN
○ Fine metal collar on tooth # _____   ○ Show no metal standard on # _____
○ Show no metal 360° on tooth # _____   ○ Porcelain Butt Margin on tooth # _____

CONTACTS
○ Broad   ○ Normal   ○ Point

OCCLUSAL CLEARANCE
○ Positive Contact   ○ Cusp Fossa   ○ Out of Occlusion   ○ Foil Relief

OCCLUSAL STAINING
○ None
○ Light
○ Medium
○ Dark
○ Hypo-calcification
○ Shade tab enclosed

MOLD OF CROWN DESIRED
○ Follow study model
○ Match existing
○ Make ideal

SURFACE ANATOMY
○ Smooth
○ Textured
○ Mamelon development
○ Match existing

PONTIC DESIGN
Harmony   Ovate   Ridge Lap
Cone   Hygienic

PONTIC TISSUE RELIEF
○ Yes mm deep _____ ○ No _____

Doctor's Signature _____ License # _____

White - Lab Copy   Yellow - Lab Copy   Blue - Doctor's Copy

Courtesy Ward Dental Laboratory, Brighton, MI.

SOFTWARE TUTORIAL

Note: Before completing the following activities, it is necessary to install the EagleSoft Demonstration disk found at the back of this workbook.

If you see a screen labeled "Patterson EagleSoft Hardware Compliance Warning" after you first start the software, this is simply a notice that you have programs running on your computer that could interfere with the running of the EagleSoft programs. Please ignore this message for now and contact support at 1-800-475-5036 if you do experience issues with the software running.

Once the program is running, change the mode in which the software will present by selecting *Window* in the main menu and clicking on *Practice Management Mode.* You are now ready to begin.

21. Complete the entry of one new provider and patient registration for three new patients with the following steps:
    a. First enter as provider Joseph W. Lake. From the menu buttons at the top of the screen, click *List,* then *Providers/ Staff,* and *New.* Enter the information below. (*Note*: If you get pop-up boxes asking whether the new zip code you entered should be added and whether you are sure that you want to continue without setting up provider hours, click *ok* and close these windows. It is recommended that you set up the provider hours using the button on the right side of the screen before moving to the next step.)

Provider

Provider ID: JWL
Name: Joseph W. Lake
Street address: 611 Main St. SE
City, state, and zip: Grand Rapids, MI 49502
Phone: 616-101-9575
Fax: 616-101-9999
E-mail: office@dapc.com
Position: Dentist

    b. When you are ready to enter patients, click on the *Person* icon in the upper left portion of the screen; then select *New* at the bottom of the screen. Insert all the patient data. Data provided below for each patient takes you logically through the prompted information on the Patterson EagleSoft screen.
    c. After completing the registration of patient 1, save the data.
    d. Return to the person screen and select *New* once again. Scroll down to patient 2 and enter the registration data. Repeat this activity for all three patients.

Patient 1
Personal Information
Name: Ms. Audra Maria Chavez
Nickname: None
Ms. Chavez is a patient, policyholder, and her own responsible party.
Street address: 11837 Belmont Rd.
City, state, zip: Ada, MI 49561
Home phone: 616-239-9999
Work phone: 616-561-7777 (no extension)
Cell phone: 616-239-1212
Marital status: Divorced
Birth date: 10/27/1962
Social Security number: 001-33-2121
Chart ID: 1156
Driver license number: C77788999
E-mail address: ca1234@dellcom.net (She would like to receive information via e-mail.)

Employment and Insurance Information
To add employment information, click on the blue underlined employer hyperlink and select *New.*

Employer:
Ace Art Supplies
1237 Auburn Ave.
Hudson, MI 49509
Phone: 1-800-444-4444

Insurance:
Group name: None
Group number: 150
Deductible: $25
Maximum benefit/year: $1000; renews each January
Company: Delta Dental of Michigan
Note: This insurance company is not in the system and must be added by clicking on the blue hyperlink Ins. Company and then on New and entering the following information:

Delta Dental of Michigan
P.O. Box 100
Littleton, MI 49509
Contact person: Jeremy Wright
Phone: 1-800-555-5555

- Click *OK* to save this data.
- Click *USE* to use this new information on the employer information.
- Click *OK* to save this new employer.
- Click *Use* to use this new employer on this patient's record.

Medical Information

The following information relates to the vertical listing of buttons on the right of the patient information.

- Enter the patient's insurance Policy holder #1300 by clicking on the *Preferences* button on the right side of the patient window. Put the number under the *Primary Member ID* field.
- Enter the patient's emergency contact by clicking on the *Prompts* button on the right side of patient window.

  Contact: Robert Chavez
  Phone number: 616-561-0011

  Click *OK* to close the prompts window.

- Select the *Med History* button to enter the following types of information; enter *Save* when information is completed. (*Note:* It helps by using the mark all *NO* feature first and then making any necessary changes before entering medical concerns.) To access the medical history information, the profile must be saved.
  - Family physician is Geraldo Gamez, DO, and patient currently under this physicians care
  - Only hospitalization or surgeries are tonsillectomy and gallbladder removal
  - Currently taking Metformin 500 mg TID
  - Has never taken Phen-Fen or Redux
  - On a low-carbohydrate diet
  - Does not use tobacco
  - Does not use controlled substances
  - Allergic to penicillin, codeine, and acrylic
  - Only health issues are type 2 diabetes and sinusitis

Charting

The *Existing Oral Conditions* are generally added to the patient tooth chart by the clinical staff. To use the clinical software, click on the image of the computer monitor with the dental chair on it on your desktop. Click on the chair to select Audra as a clinical patient. There are several charting methods in use by computer systems; to switch to the charting method explained in the text, go to *File → Preferences →* click on *Chart* tab *→* check *Use Solid Fill →* click *OK*. Next select the *Chart* module by clicking on the cupboard door panel that is labeled *Chart* and then selecting and double-clicking on your patient's name.

Charting Existing Oral Conditions

Note: To chart on a tooth, you must click on it. Conditions appear as abbreviations on the buttons along the right side of the screen. If you need to see additional information to determine what an abbreviation means, roll your cursor over that button without clicking it.

Tooth No.	Condition
1, 16, and 17	Missing (*Missing* button on right)
3	MO amalgam (*AMAL* button; be sure to mark existing and surfaces.)
5	DO composite (*COMPp*)
8	MI composite (*COM A*)
14	PFM
20	MOD composite (*COMPp*)
24 and 25	Root canals (RCT) with PFM crowns (*ENDO* button)
31	MODL amalgam that is defective

Entering Proposed Treatment

Follow the same steps listed above, but ensure that each service is marked as *proposed*.

Tooth No.	Condition
27	Class V composite
31	PFM crown

46

To record services that are not tooth specific, simply click on that specific service button on the right of the screen without selecting a tooth first.

- Prophylaxis needed
- 4 black and white radiographs
- 2 PA radiographs; teeth 24 and 25 and 31 and 32 (found on the drop-down arrow next to *BWX4*). Note that there is a separate code for the additional PA x-ray.
  Save this information before leaving this window.

Patient 2

Basic Information

Name: Mr. Edward Raymond
Nickname: Ed
Mr. Raymond is a patient and responsible party.
Street address: 1978 Woodwind Dr.
City, state, zip: Bedford, MI 49508
Home phone: 616-990-0099
Work phone: 616-561-2222 (no extension)
Cell phone: 616-239-3334
Marital status: Married
Birth date: 05/05/1938
Social Security number: 009-00-2121
Chart ID: 1923
Driver license number: R4950999
E-mail address: er1234@belleast.com

Employment and Insurance Information

Employment: Retired
Insurance: None (Do not mark the policy holder option.)

Additional Information

Emergency contact: Phyllis Raymond (spouse); 616-239-0022
Medical history:

- Under physician's care; post-liver transplant; physician: Mark Harrington, MD
- Liver transplant operation in 2001
- Medications: tacrolimus, atenolol, warfarin
- Allergies to penicillin, latex, intravenous contrast dye
- Conditions: anemia, gout, blood transfusion, high blood pressure, liver disease, rheumatic fever, shingles
- Serious illness: primary sclerosing cholangitis

Charting

Charting Existing Oral Conditions

Tooth No.	Condition
1, 16, 17, and 32	Missing
2	MOD amalgam
3	Decay MO
4	O Composite
5	MO composite
9	MI composite
10	M composite
15	PFM
19	Buccal class V composite
20	Buccal class V composite
21	MOD composite
24	Fractured MI angle (use detailed surfaces)
30	MODL amalgam that is fractured

Entering Proposed Treatment

Tooth No.	Condition
3	MO composite
24	MI composite
30	PFM crown

- Tooth whitening
- Prophylaxis needed
- Four black and white radiographs

Patient 3

Personal Information

Name: Mrs. Catherine Gordon
Nickname: Kate
Mrs. Gordon is the patient, policyholder, and responsible party.
Street address:18841 Grand Isles Lane
City, state, zip: Grand Rapids, MI 49508
Home phone: 616-390-0099
Work phone: 616-561-4443
Cell phone: 616-239-1924
Marital status: Married
Birth date: 02/10/1942
Social Security number: 999-00-3131
Chart ID: 1334
Driver license number: G34021939
E-mail address: kmg4321@belleast.com

Employment and Insurance Information

Employer: World Color Press (This employer is already in the system.)
Insurance information: Aetna Life and Casualty (This insurance company is already in the system.)

Medical Information

Emergency contact: Mark Benjamin; 616-239-5454
Policy holder: 1200
Medical history:

- Under physician's care; allergy desensitization; family physician: Cynthia Huckins, MD
- Hospitalized: childbirth ×4
- Medications: lisinopril, albuterol inhaler
- Allergies: trees, dust mites
- Conditions: asthma, high blood pressure, shingles
- No serious illness

Charting

Charting Existing Oral Conditions

Tooth No.	Condition
1, 32	Missing
2	MOD onlay
3	Decay DO
4	MO Composite
6	MO composite
8 and 9	MI composite
15	PFM
19	Buccal Class V composite
20	Buccal Class V composite
21	MOD composite
23, 24, 25, 26	Missing
22	MODL composite, fractured
27	O amalgam
30	MODL amalgam that is fractured

48

Entering Proposed Treatment

Tooth No.	Condition
3	MO composite
23, 24, 25, 26	PFM pontics
22 and 27	PFM crowns as bridge abutments.
29	MO composite
30	PFM crown

- Tooth whitening
- Prophylaxis needed
- Four black and white radiographs

CRITICAL THINKING ACTIVITY

Consider how you could save time using a computer charting system rather than a manual system with symbols. What would be the disadvantages of using a computer charting system? What would be the advantages to the office and to the patient?

8 Storage of Business Records

With the vast amounts of information generated in the dental office and not all dental offices in a paperless modality, reality dictates that traditional methods of record storage must be used. The administrative staff is responsible for managing and maintaining both paper and electronic files. This chapter discusses records storage and provides helpful information about making this daunting task more palatable. Review the material in this chapter, and become familiar with the basic systems used for document storage. Then complete the materials in this chapter of the workbook to ensure that you will become an efficient manager of records storage in the dental office where you are employed.

LEARNING OUTCOMES

On completion of the text and workbook chapters, the student should be able to do the following:
- Define key terms.
- Identify and distinguish among the different storage systems.
- Apply basic alphabetic indexing rules.
- Determine the most efficient storage methods for various documents in a dental office.
- Select supplies for the storage of records.

SHORT-ANSWER OR FILL-IN QUESTIONS

1. List and describe the basic steps one should follow in preparing to file any type of documents.

_____

_____

_____

_____

_____

_____

_____

_____

_____

_____

_____

2. Match the term in Column A with the definition in Column B that best describes the term.

	Column A	**Column B**
_____	Cross-referencing	a. Stores records in drawers that pull out
_____	Retrieval	b. Follow-up file
_____	Open-shelf filing	c. Similar to a vertical file, except the longest side opens as if records were placed on a bookshelf
_____	Lateral file	d. Aids in fast retrieval and refiling
_____	Vertical file	e. The removal of records from files using proper "charge-out" methods
_____	Tickler file	f. Usually heavy cardboard; divides the file drawer into separate sections
_____	File guides	g. Similar to lateral file but with no doors to close
_____	Color-coding	h. Alerts staff members that a record normally kept in a specific location has been stored elsewhere

MULTIPLE-CHOICE QUESTIONS

3. A new filing system for clinical charts is to be installed in the office. Which of the following would be most efficient?
   a. Open files with colored filing labels with alpha and numeric codes
   b. Vertical files with tabbed-top labels
   c. Vertical files with closed-end folders
   d. Lateral files with closed-end folders

4. From the following list of names, which of the following would be filed first and which would be filed last in alphabetic order?
   1. Harold O. Smith
   2. Richard Smythe
   3. Ronald Smythe
   4. Rick Smith
   5. Ricardo M. Smith
   a. 1 and 3
   b. 2 and 4
   c. 1 and 5
   d. 2 and 5
   e. 1 and 4

5. From the following list of dental supply companies, which of the following would be filed first and which would be filed last in alphabetic order?
   1. Davis and Davis Laboratory
   2. Quick Copy
   3. Apex Dental Supplies
   4. Albert D. Apple Laboratory
   5. QT Surgical Supply
   a. 1 and 2
   b. 3 and 5
   c. 4 and 2
   d. 4 and 5

6. An electronic code at the bottom of a document includes the following data:

   Caledonia/Phillips/Letter/Resf.MJRadick

   It is likely that the second listing is the:
   a. office location.
   b. originator.
   c. directory name.
   d. document name.

7. A file that is used to include items to be completed in the future is referred to as a/an:
    a. chronologic system.
    b. alpha system.
    c. numeric system.
    d. tickler file.

PRACTICAL ACTIVITIES

8. Assume that the following list of names, with addresses, represents a contact list of business or companies commonly used by the practice. (*Note:* If using a computer, sort the names first in alphabetic order and second in a geographic file in order by state and then by cities in the state.)

Apex Dental Supplies
1816 S. Riverfront
Elgin, IL 26582

T. S. Davis
26058 S. State
Chicago, IL 26528
Quality Instruments
P.O. Box D-1
Minneapolis, MN 48807

J. P. T. Uniforms
22803 Third Avenue
Benton Harbor, MI 23062

Davis & Davis Office Supplies
4800 N. Baseline
Grand Rapids, MI 27501

M & M Creative Systems
11015 Orange Avenue
Los Angeles, CA 90025

Albert D. Apple
3668 N.W. Territorial
Buffalo, NY 32506

Quick Copy
1108 Third Street
Des Moines, IA 42106

QT Surgical Supplies
1556 Eighth Street SW
Dubuque, IA 42013

Robert S. Davis, C.P.A.
90724 S. Hubbard
Gary, IN 30682

Mark C. Sylvester
2601 Beck Boulevard
Albany, NY 30582

Telcom Credit Bureau
914 E. Michigan
Madison, WI 78034

C. V. Talbot
2247 Hamilton
Charleston, WV 82506

Talbot & Associates
839 Frederick
Hampton, VA 26809

B B Waste Paper Co.
1308 Cadillac
Charlotte, NC 89045

Brian Baumgartner
6262 Shield
Jamestown, ND 45902

Consumer Counseling
590 Bridge Street
Charleston, SC 78032

E. S. Comstock
1255 Harbour Cove
Los Altos, CA 91256

Community Pharmacy
2236 Stadium Drive
Kansas City, MO 64119

Krauss & Krauss Drugs, Inc.
152 Barkber Boulevard
Kansas City, KS 78566

Davis and Bradshaw Laboratories
5697 West Beltline Dr.
Grand Rapids, MI 49506

9. The following listings of names represent patients' files to be used for a marketing project.
   a. Prepare a list showing the first, second, third, and, where applicable, the fourth indexing units. (*Hint:* This could be done in Word as a table or in another program such as Excel or Access. If you have not done a table in Word, go to *Help* and follow the basic instructions.)
   b. With the same list of names, prepare an alphabetic listing as the names would appear in an alphabetic file.
   c. The patients' names also have an account number. Prepare a second listing of these names by number as they would appear in a numeric file (number followed by name).
   d. Merge List B with List A, and prepare a new listing of patients' names as they would appear in the alphabetic file. Provide the final list with the following: surname, first name, middle initial or name, and case number.

List A

Phyllis Prestock	10005	Stephen Carole	10013
Mary Martin	10002	G. R. Anderson	10006
Nora Nummy	10009	Johnathan Reiker	10033
Donna Turnbolt	10044	Kathryn Geer	10007
Maria Hehir	10012	G. Robert Andersen	10040
John Maxey Jr.	10046	J. T. Schmidt	10029
Oahn Ho	10011	Andrea Voitik	10015
Mary J. Martin	10026	Morris Edwards	10045
Stanley Ferry	10021	Shirley Utz	11003
John Goodman	10031	Peter Utz	11023
Hong Viu	10035		
J. J. Goble	10047		
Jesu Ricca	10041	**List B**	
Philip Hansen	10014	Henry Corrigan	10175
Patricia Dixon	10023	Mary Jane Allemeir	10090
Mark Hopkins	10020	Michael Jensen	10190
Ralph Fletcher	10036	Mary Louise Puchaski	10116
Nellie Trowbaum	10030	Joseph Cavero	10119
Amy Goble	10042	Rosa Cortes	10097
Phil Hansen	10047	Henry Strohs	10082
Mary Richards	10003	Sally McBee	10114
Richard Shilling	10019	Jed Thompson	10046
Adam C. Fields	10001	Trudy Desrosiers	10074
Gertrude Teiber	10010	Sally Ferez	10192
Ralph Parker	10034	Paul Douglas	10064
Leonard Kuhn	10022	Alice Thomas	10071
Stephanie Carroll	10032	Mary Jo Flemming	10068
Walter Busch	10008	James LuNardelli	10143
Dale Noeker	10050	Robert Lunde	10189
Frieda Graves	10028	S. B. Porter	10092
Harold G. Hammond	10024	S. B. Darrett	10058
Richard Schwartz	10016	Sam Grigsby	10199
Tina Reese	10037	Charles Saint John	10089
Martin Reddick	10027	Mark L. Puchaski	10074
Susan Sasman	10043	Brian S. Porter	10116
Debbie Jones	10049	Cliff McBride	10057
Fred Stanley	10025	Michele Havlichek	10096
Roger Nichols	10039	Charles St. Johns	10091
G. Harold Hamond	10038		
Phillip Rhodes	10017		

CRITICAL THINKING ACTIVITY

There seems to be a constant problem with paper clinical records being lost or mislaid. The doctor seldom takes records out of the office, but when she does there is no indication where that particular record goes. The dental hygienist returns all patient records to the business office at the end of the working day. You use a date and letter system that identifies each record. Other than the one indication by the doctor, no one on the staff is willing to accept responsibility for this constant problem. What might be a way that you could meet and resolve this problem?

9 Written Communications

Written communication in all of its forms remains extremely important. In addition to e-mail, the administrative assistant will use instant messaging via the Internet and write memorandums, letters, and reports. Effective written correspondence promotes goodwill for the office, whereas ineffectively written correspondence can cost the dental office greatly in unhappy patients and goodwill.

The administrative assistant must be able to produce professionally written documents that sound like a person speaking to another person. In addition, the assistant must be aware of basic rules of written communication and be thorough and accurate in producing all forms of written communication. After reviewing the textbook chapter, complete the questions and activities in this workbook chapter to ensure that you are able to put into practice the basic rules of written communication that will present a professional image for the office, be highly accurate, and be easily understood by the reader.

LEARNING OUTCOMES

On completion of text and workbook chapters, the student should be able to do the following:
- Define key terms.
- Describe the various types of written communication in a dental office.
- Select stationery supplies.
- Identify the characteristics of effective correspondence.
- Identify the parts of a letter.
- Review rules of punctuation and capitalization.
- Describe the basic steps for preparing written communication.
- Apply various formatting styles to written communication.
- Describe standard procedures for preparing outgoing mail.
- Observe ethical and legal obligations in written communication.
- Explain the use of e-mail in the dental office.
- Apply common business etiquette to the use of e-mail.
- Identify the classifications of mail.
- Identify special mail services.
- Explain the function of a postage meter.
- Discuss the process for packaging laboratory cases.
- Explain the procedure for sorting incoming mail.

SHORT-ANSWER OR FILL-IN QUESTIONS

1. Identify five types of written communication that are used in a dental office.

   1. _____

   2. _____

   3. _____

   4. _____

   5. _____

57

2. Describe six characteristics of an effective letter.

1. _____

2. _____

3. _____

4. _____

5. _____

6. _____

3. Name and explain the parts of a business letter.

_____

_____

_____

_____

_____

_____

_____

_____

4. You are writing to the governor of the state in which you live about an issue with the state dental practice act. How would you address the letter? What is the name of the governor of your state? What is the complete address that you would use? Where can you find this information?

_____

_____

_____

_____

5. You are writing to the president of a state university. How would you address the letter? What would be the salutation? Where would you find the president's address?

_____

_____

_____

_____

_____

_____

6. How should the name and address appear if you are writing to Dr. Kimberly Thompson, who is a DDS and whose address is 12568 Upper Sandusky Ave., Caledonia, MI 49509?

_____

_____

_____

7. What are the nine basic steps to follow in writing a letter?

1. _____

2. _____

3. _____

4. _____

5. _____

6. _____

7. _____

8. _____

9. _____

8. Identify and describe five different classifications of mail.

1. _____

   _____

2. _____

   _____

3. _____

   _____

4. _____

   _____

5. _____

   _____

MATCHING EXERCISE

9. Match the punctuation mark in Column A with the description in Column B.

	Column A	**Column B**
_____	Period	a. Used after the salutation in a business letter
_____	Comma	b. Used ordinarily after words or groups of words that express command, strong feeling, emotion
_____	Semicolon	c. Used between independent groups or clauses that are long or that contain parts that are separated by commas
_____	Colon	d. Used to indicate possession
_____	Exclamation point	e. Indicates a partial stop and separates coordinate clauses that are connected by conjunctions
_____	Dash	f. Used to indicate an omission of letters or figures or to cause a definite stop in reading the letter
_____	Apostrophe	g. Indicates a full stop and is used at the end of a complete declarative or imperative sentence

MULTIPLE-CHOICE QUESTIONS

10. Which of the following sentences is grammatically correct?
    a. Me and Tony went to the dental laboratory last week for a tour.
    b. Tony and me went to the dental laboratory last week for a tour.
    c. Tony and I went to the dental laboratory last week for a tour.

11. Which of the following sentences is not grammatically correct?
    a. Its probably going to take longer to complete the treatment.
    b. It's probably going to take longer to complete the treatment.

12. Which of the following sentences has a misspelled word?
    a. The stool seems stationery.
    b. We need to order three boxes of stationery.
    c. The new position of the chair is stationary.

13. Which of the following sentences has incorrect punctuation?
    a. The Taylors' records need to be transferred to a new dentist.
    b. The Taylor's records need to be transferred to a new dentist.
    c. The Taylors will not be returning to the practice.

14. If you use spell-check on a computer software system, you can be assured that all words in a letter will be spelled correctly.
    a. True
    b. False

15. The U.S. Postal Service (USPS) recommends that punctuation be eliminated on envelope addresses.
    a. True
    b. False

16. Which of the following is the typical order of a business letter?
    a. Date line, inside address, reference initials, salutation, body of letter, complimentary close, keyed signature
    b. Inside address, date line, salutation, body of letter, complimentary close, keyed signature
    c. Date line, inside address, salutation, body of letter, complimentary close, keyed signature, reference initials
    d. Date line, inside address, salutation, body of letter, complimentary close, reference initials, keyed signature

17. With the use of word processing and graphics software, it is possible to eliminate the purchase of preprinted stationery.
    a. True
    b. False

18. The doctor reviews a letter that contains the following paragraph and indicates that it has several errors. How many errors are in the following paragraph?

    The patient was seen for a prophylaxes but due to her physical ability she couldn't keep her mouth open long enough for deep scaleing. Her mothers assistance was a grate help to the hygenist.

    a. Two
    b. Three
    c. Four
    d. Five

19. Which of the following sentences has a misspelled word?
    a. The occlusal surface is to be restored.
    b. The periapicale region is sensitive.
    c. The orthodontist will see her next week.
    d. The periodontist is out of town this week.

20. Which of the following sentences has a misspelled word?
    a. The reconciliation was done earlier.
    b. The MSDS form was incomplete.
    c. The tooth is nonsucedaneous.
    d. There is an odontoma presnt.

21. Which of the following sentences is grammatically correct?
    a. I and Dr. Wallace were at the meeting.
    b. The doctor and me attended the first seminar.
    c. The hygienist and I were among the first guests.
    d. The new patients record is on my desk.

PRACTICE WITH GRAMMAR

The list below contains a variety of statements with common grammatical errors. Rewrite the sentence in the space below as it should be corrected.

22. Me and Tony went to the dental laboratory last week for a tour.

_____

23. I seen the patient record on the desk.

_____

24. Her and I are both chairside assistants.

_____

25. I don't want no more.

_____

26. I had not known no one like that before.

_____

27. He ain't bad if you are patient with him.

_____

28. We done the sterilization before lunch time.

_____

29. They wasn't suppose to be here until this afternoon.

_____

30. She did not follow my advise.

_____

31. She sighted the correct reference.

_____

32. Its probably going to take longer to complete the treatment.

_____

33. The family had it's records transferred to this office.

_____

34. Order three boxes of stationary.

_____

35. The stool seems stationery.

_____

36. Who shall I ask first?

_____

PRACTICAL ACTIVITIES

37. In this activity you are asked to write a series of letters. Before beginning, you should create two templates and store them as *Letter template Joseph W. Lake letter* and *Interoffice memorandum template Joseph W. Lake*. You may create any type of template and are encouraged to use a graphic that is simple but professional. Use the vital office information from one of the letterheads for Dental Associates in the chapter.

    Depending on your need for experience, you may be directed by your instructor to create envelopes. These will need to be provided by you or the instructor. These letters also could be transmitted as an attachment via e-mail. If you have never created envelopes on your printer, it is wise to do so for the practice. Be certain that you review printer instructors for insertion of the envelope in the correct position.

    Addressing the envelope is fairly easy in Microsoft Word; you simply block the address, go to *Tools,* select *Envelope,* and then insert the return address and print the envelope. Try it if you have not done it before. If you do not have Microsoft Word, be certain to familiarize yourself with the procedure using your software.

    The following letters have been directed to be written by Dr. Lake, and the assistant is named Jennifer Ellis. You may substitute your own name in the place of Jennifer Ellis if you prefer.

    When finished you should have the following assignments completed:

- Letter to Mrs. Jason Calloway
- Letter to Reliance Dental Laboratory
- Letter to Mr. Robert Clay
- Second page of a letter to James Howard, DDS
- Letter to Joseph E. Harrison, DDS, for Mr. Howard Phillips
- Letter to Jack Notman, DDS
- Rekeyed and corrected letter

Letter 1

Keyboard the following letter in block style with mixed punctuation. Use the current date and address a small envelope, if available. Fold the letter to insert into a small envelope. Make a copy for the office files or store it electronically.

Mrs. Jason Calloway, 2453 Prescott Avenue, Grandville, MI 49302 Dear Mrs. Calloway (P) We have written to Doctor Jack Notman as you requested. He is most interested in your case and will be expecting you to contact his office very soon. (P) When we first corresponded with Doctor Notman, we mailed him a complete set of radiographs. Also, we indicated to him at that time that you are a diabetic and have allergies to several drugs. (P) As soon as time is available for Doctor Notman to complete the work, I suggest you contact his office. If we can be of further assistance, do not hesitate to call us. Sincerely Joseph W. Lake, D.D.S. (reference initials)

Letter 2

Keyboard the following letter in modified block style with open punctuation. Use the current date and address a large envelope, if available. Fold the letter to insert into a large envelope. Make a copy for the office files or store it electronically.

Reliance Dental Laboratory, 1600 Michigan Avenue, NE, Grand Rapids, MI 49502 Gentlemen (Subject line: Three-Unit Porcelain-Fused-to-Metal Bridge); (P) I am returning the three-unit porcelain-fused-to-metal bridge you constructed for our patient, Mr. H.B. Rider. There are open margins on teeth #9 on the mesial, #10 on the facial, and #11 on the distal. (P) I am mailing a new final impression that can be used for recasting of the bridge. I would like the bridge returned with the castings only soldered in place for a try-in. If the bridge is satisfactory, I will return the casting for final baking of the porcelain. (P) We appreciate your cooperation in this matter. Sincerely, Joseph W. Lake, D.D.S. (reference initials)

Letter 3

Keyboard the following letter in block style with mixed punctuation. Use the current date and an appropriate-size envelope, if available. Make a copy for the office files or store it electronically.

Mr. Robert Clay, 6690 Jefferson SW, Wyoming, MI 49507 Dear Mr. Clay (P) I know you have been pleased with the work our office has done for you and your wife. We have enjoyed having both of you as patients. (P) We feel sure you have misplaced the last two statements that we have sent to you, but we would appreciate it if you would stop by the office so we can make an arrangement to bring your account up-to-date. (P) Thank you for your cooperation in this matter. Sincerely, Jennifer Ellis, R.D.A.

Letter 4

Keyboard the following information as the continuation of a two-page letter, and use blank stationery. The letter has been addressed to James Howard, DDS. Use modified block style and open punctuation. Make a copy for the office files or store it electronically. Make an additional copy to be sent to O.J. Fox, DDS.

(P)To confirm an almost conclusive diagnosis, we are referring the patient to you for an incisional biopsy. The biopsy was not done in our office due to the potential hemorrhage problem. If my diagnosis of squamous cell carcinoma is confirmed, we recommend counseling to the patient so that treatment can begin immediately. (P) If we can be of further assistance, please feel free to contact our office. Sincerely, Joseph W. Lake, D.D.S. (reference initials)

Letter 5

Keyboard a patient referral letter to Joseph E. Harrison, DDS, MS, 1718 West Stadium Boulevard, Ann Arbor, MI 48104. Compose a letter using the following information taken from the patient's clinical chart:

The patient is Howard Phillips, age 37. Tooth #32 is to be removed. The patient prefers general anesthesia. His health history indicates that he has had rheumatic fever and is under the care of Mark Driscoll, M.D. at 211 Cutler Street SW, Grand Rapids, MI 49507. A periapical x-ray of this area is to be included. Keyboard the letter in modified block style, use the current date, make a copy, address an appropriate envelope, and have the letter available for Dr. Lake's signature.

Letter 6

The administrative assistant may write many letters using his or her own personal signature. The following note appears on your desk from Dr. Lake:

> Jennifer:
> Would you please write to Dr. Notman (Jack) and ask him to return the few books I loaned him on Practice Administration and Evaluation? I need these for reference for the seminar I am presenting to the Council on Dental Practice. .
>
> Let him know that he is most willing to borrow them again as soon as I get some notes from them.
>
> Thanks,
> Dr. Lake

Dr. Notman's address appears in your address file as follows: Jack Notman, D.D.S., 255 W. Michigan, Grand Rapids, MI 49501.

Letter 7

The letter on p. 65 contains errors. Proofread the letter and make corrections in spelling and punctuation. Rekey the letter using office stationery with block format and mixed punctuation, including today's date. Address an appropriate envelope. Make a copy for the office files or store it electronically.

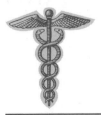

Dental Associates, PC
Joseph W. Lake, DDS – Ashley M. Lake, DDS

March 12, 20___

Mark Stevens D.D.S., M.S.
2346 Plaza Way
Grandville, MI 48903

Dear Dr. Stevens,

As a follow up to our telephone conversation of March 9th, I would like to introduce, Skip Frederick, for an examination and referral. He is a thirty-seven-year-old male who has a chief complaint of pain in the left side of his mandible. The onset of his pain was four weeks ago during a meal. While chewing he felt a pop or click in his jaw. At first he thought it was his tempromandibular joint, but later he noticed the pain in the midbody of the mandible.

His past medical history reveals that he has a grade IV systolic heart murmur, a hyatal hernia and a family history of osteogenesis imperfecta. He takes Prilosec and antacids and also receives antibiotic prophylacsis before dental treatment. He has no known allergies. As a child he was hospitalized for arm and leg fractures.

Complete mouth radiographs reveal impacted third molars, mild bone loss around his maxillary and mandibular molars and a fractured amalgam on the mandibular left first molar (#18). An oral examination confirms mild periodontitis and the fractured amalgam. Other noteworthy findings include Class III mobility of #18 and 'electric shock like pain' that radiates to his lower lip when he clenches his teeth. His radiographs are enclosed. Please evaluate and treat as necessary including the removal of his third molars.

I appreciate your time and consideration. Please let me know the diagnosis and treatment plan.

Very truly yours,

Ashley M. Lake, DDS

611 Main Street, SE – Grand Rapids, MI 49502   Phone: 616.101.9575 Fax: 616.101.9999
E-mail: office@dapc.com or Visit us at: www.Lakedental.com

38. Assume that the following list represents the morning incoming mail. How would you sort and handle each item?
   a. Product advertisement and sample of a new composite material for Drs. Ashley and Joseph Lake

   _____

   b. Letter addressed to Dr. Ashley Lake marked *Personal*

   _____

   c. Letter addressed to the administrative assistant regarding overpayment of an account

   _____

   d. Statement of account from Quick Copy

   _____

   e. Check in the amount of $850.00 from Harold C. Hammond (a patient)

   _____

   f. Two magazines, *The American Dental Association Journal* and *Reader's Digest,* addressed to Dental Associates

   _____

   g. Notice of a registered letter for Dr. Joseph Lake at the post office

   _____

   h. OSHA *Update Newsletter* marked *Important Dated Material*

   _____

   i. Concert tickets for Dr. Ashley Lake

   _____

   j. Notice of Dental Assistant Advisory Committee meeting from Kent County Community College for Dr. Ashley Lake

   _____

   k. Two statements, one each to Dr. Joseph and Dr. Ashley Lake, for Kent County District Dental Society dues

   _____

   l. Letter to Dr. Joseph Lake from Rotary Club confirming a speaking engagement

   _____

39. The following list represents the outgoing mail for the office. Indicate how you would prepare each item for mailing. (Indicate any special handling or delivery services.)
- Letter and statement to a patient (You want proof of its delivery.)

_____

- Pamphlet weighing 12 oz

_____

- Completed manuscript to a publisher weighing 18 oz

_____

- Recall notices to 30 patients

_____

- Package weighing 10 lb, valued at $550.00

_____

- Package delivered to the office that Dr. Lake refuses to accept

_____

- Laboratory requisition with impressions and ancillary materials for a porcelain veneer crown that is to be sent to Nuva Dent Porcelain Laboratory, 819 West 43rd Street, New York, NY 67845. This item must be insured for $500.00.

_____

- A letter and a CD with radiographs to be mailed locally to a periodontist

_____

- DVD to be returned for credit to a distributor in Chicago, IL 60611

_____

CRITICAL THINKING ACTIVITY

Describe the difference in the fold of an envelope for a standard business envelope versus a small envelope. What is an alternative fold for a business envelope? Have you tried these folds? Did you know that when you open a letter, the inside address should be immediately visible and the reader should not have to turn the letter around to read the top of the letter?

INTERNET ASSIGNMENT

Go to www.usps.gov and www.fedex.com and observe the various types of services that are provided by these two groups. Determine which method would be the most economical transport of a case from your office to a dental laboratory in Upper Saddle, NJ.

10 | Telecommunications

A revolution is taking place in the field of telecommunications. Trying to keep up with the latest devices in telecommunications is like trying to keep up with all the new brands of composite restorative materials in clinical dentistry. It is up to the administrative assistant in a busy dental office to complete the research on the most current models and to determine the application of the latest telecommunications technology for the office.

It is critical that the administrative assistant be familiar with changes in technology and able to maintain current telecommunications in the dental office. Modern telecommunications is now the most important communication system in the world because it is perhaps the fastest and easiest way to transmit messages. Therefore the administrative assistant must assume responsibility for ensuring that the staff is well informed about the use of the telecommunications systems in the office and able to present a good image for the office when using these systems. Review the materials in the textbook chapter, and then complete the questions and activities in this chapter of the workbook to ensure a thorough understanding of the use of telecommunications in the dental office.

LEARNING OUTCOMES

On completion of text and workbook chapters, the student should be able to do the following:
- Define key terms.
- Explain the application of telecommunications in a dental office.
- Describe various types of telecommunication systems commonly used by the dental team.
- Practice efficient telephone techniques.
- Receive, transmit, and record telephone messages.
- Plan and place outgoing telephone calls.
- Describe cell phone rules of etiquette.
- Describe the use of text messaging.
- Use the features of special telephone equipment and services.
- Describe the best way to manage telephone calls commonly encountered in the dental office.

SHORT-ANSWER OR FILL-IN QUESTIONS

1. List and briefly describe eight various types of information that can be found in a telephone directory.

    1. _____

    2. _____

    3. _____

    4. _____

    5. _____

    6. _____

    7. _____

    8. _____

2. Locate telephone numbers for each of the following. Keyboard the names and telephone numbers in tabular format on a Rolodex-type form provided in the classroom or the office of employment.

a. Internal Revenue Service

_____

_____

b. Police department (non-emergency number)

_____

_____

c. U.S. post office

_____

_____

d. State employment commission

_____

_____

3. Using the Yellow Pages, locate one company and telephone number for each of the following. Record the information on a Rolodex form provided in the classroom or the office of employment.

a. Dental supply company

_____

_____

b. Dental laboratory

_____

_____

c. Computer repair service

_____

_____

d. Pharmacy

_____

_____

4. You receive the following calls. Use the telephone message forms provided below to write down the appropriate message. Complete the information about each call and sign your name.

a. Dr. Lake's wife calls at 9:30 AM and asks you to remind him that he is to stop at Great Lake's Bank to pick up the mortgage forms on his way home today.

TO _____

DATE _____ TIME _____

WHILE YOU WERE OUT

M_____

of_____

Phone No._____

TELEPHONED		PLEASE CALL
WAS IN TO SEE YOU		WILL CALL BACK
WANTS TO SEE YOU		**URGENT**
RETURNED YOUR CALL		

Message _____

_____

_____

_____

_____

Operator _____

b. Mr. Horace Schramm calls at 10:10 AM to remind Dr. Lake that a special meeting of the administration council has been scheduled for 4:00 PM tomorrow.

TO _____

DATE _____ TIME _____

WHILE YOU WERE OUT

M_____

of_____

Phone No._____

TELEPHONED		PLEASE CALL
WAS IN TO SEE YOU		WILL CALL BACK
WANTS TO SEE YOU		**URGENT**
RETURNED YOUR CALL		

Message _____

_____

_____

_____

_____

Operator _____

c. Mr. Daniel Rogers calls at 10:40 AM and wants to discuss the sale of some property. He will be leaving the office at noon and will not return until after 3:00 PM today. His number is 271-3364.

```
TO _____

DATE _____ TIME _____

        WHILE YOU WERE OUT

M_____

of_____

Phone No._____
┌─────────────────────┬─────────────────────┐
│ TELEPHONED          │ PLEASE CALL         │
├─────────────────────┼─────────────────────┤
│ WAS IN TO SEE YOU   │ WILL CALL BACK      │
├─────────────────────┼─────────────────────┤
│ WANTS TO SEE YOU    │                     │
├─────────────────────┤     URGENT          │
│ RETURNED YOUR CALL  │                     │
└─────────────────────┴─────────────────────┘

Message _____
_____
_____
_____
_____

        Operator _____
```

d. Mrs. Tod Rae calls at 11:00 AM, upset about her account. She insists on talking to the dentist before he goes to lunch. She refuses to discuss the matter with you. Her phone number is 377-4721.

```
TO _____

DATE _____ TIME _____

        WHILE YOU WERE OUT

M_____

of_____

Phone No._____
┌─────────────────────┬─────────────────────┐
│ TELEPHONED          │ PLEASE CALL         │
├─────────────────────┼─────────────────────┤
│ WAS IN TO SEE YOU   │ WILL CALL BACK      │
├─────────────────────┼─────────────────────┤
│ WANTS TO SEE YOU    │                     │
├─────────────────────┤     URGENT          │
│ RETURNED YOUR CALL  │                     │
└─────────────────────┴─────────────────────┘

Message _____
_____
_____
_____
_____

        Operator _____
```

5. The dentist asks you to arrange her trip to the national meeting of the American Dental Association in San Francisco. She wants to travel by the most economical fare. She needs to arrive by noon on July 18 and must return home by early evening on July 23. In a narrative form, explain what you would do and type an itinerary for the trip.

_____

_____

_____

_____

_____

6. Identify words or phrases that might replace the following terms to create a more positive image.

Pain _____

Cancellation _____

Waiting room _____

Filling _____

My girl _____

Cost _____

Pull _____

Spit _____

Remind _____

Check-up _____

Grind the tooth; drill _____

Convention _____

The doctor is tied up _____

Nope _____

Uh huh; yep _____

Okey dokey _____

Old patient _____

Check-up _____

Price _____

7. Identify six characteristics that might be considered for a telephone in a dental office.

   1. _____

   2. _____

   3. _____

   4. _____

   5. _____

   6. _____

8. List and explain the steps one should follow when placing a person on hold to answer another call.

   _____

   _____

   _____

   _____

   _____

   _____

9. Identify 10 ideas that could be used to improve telephone etiquette for incoming and outgoing calls.

   1. _____

   2. _____

   3. _____

   4. _____

   5. _____

   6. _____

   7. _____

   8. _____

   9. _____

   10. _____

10. Which of the following is the approximate percentage of patients who enter a dental practice via the telephone?
    a. 50%
    b. 75%
    c. 80%
    d. 90%

11. Which of the following phrases should be avoided during telecommunications with patients?
    a. This won't hurt.
    b. You are making a wise investment.
    c. We will need to use a no. 17 instrument.
    d. The doctor is with a patient.

12. Which of the following words provides patient comfort?
    a. Spit
    b. Pull
    c. Cut
    d. Old patient
    e. Former patient

13. A patient contacts the office and is upset. After identifying himself, he shouts to you, "I just received my statement. It is awfully high! You must have made a mistake. I am not going to pay this much!" You should react by doing which of the following?
    a. Telling the patient that he must be wrong because you know that you did not make a mistake
    b. Telling the patient that you are going to put him on hold until he calms down
    c. Thanking the patient for calling with the concern and ask whether you could get out the record, review it, and call him back within a specified time
    d. Telling him that you are too busy now but will look it up and if it is wrong send him a new statement

14. When calling to confirm an appointment, you should announce yourself by saying what?
    a. This is Dr. Smith's office calling.
    b. This is Mary from Dr. Smith's office.
    c. Hi, this is Mary.
    d. This is Mary from the office.

15. When calling to confirm an appointment, the best statement you could use is which of the following statements?
    a. I am calling to remind you of the appointment on ….
    b. I am calling to tell you that you have an appointment on ….
    c. I am calling to confirm your appointment on ….
    d. I am calling to see whether you can still keep your appointment on ….

16. The office from which you are making a long-distance call is in Virginia. You are calling a dental manufacturer in Spokane, Washington. The office you are calling opens at 10:00 AM. What is the earliest time you could make the call from Virginia to ensure that the office will be open?
    a. 10:00 AM
    b. 11:00 AM
    c. 1:00 PM
    d. 2:00 PM

CRITICAL THINKING ACTIVITIES

1. A patient has an outstanding account in your office. You phone the home, but there is no answer and no answering machine. You call the patient at work, and a co-worker answers the telephone. He asks whether he could take a message. You inform him that you want this patient to call you back about her delinquent account in your office. You give him your name and telephone number. What are the ramifications of the action you took in this situation?

2. You send a fax with complete patient information on it to another professional office and do not send a cover sheet. What is the impact of this action? How could you have avoided a problem situation?

Appointment Management Systems

Appointment management in today's dental practice most often takes the form of a software system. The traditional appointment book, although still available, is used less frequently but is still presented in this chapter because the concepts of scheduling apply to both the manual and appointment scheduling software systems installed in the office computer. Appointment management on the computer is a primary responsibility of the administrative assistant and can be the key to a productive practice. After reviewing the materials in the textbook chapter, complete the activities in this workbook chapter to ensure complete understanding of the concepts of appointment management.

LEARNING OUTCOMES

On completion of text and workbook chapters, the student should be able to do the following:
- Define key terms.
- Describe appointment book styles.
- Describe appointment software options.
- Complete an appointment matrix.
- Identify solutions to common appointment scheduling problems.
- Make an appointment entry.
- Design an appointment schedule list.
- Identify common appointment book symbols.
- Describe the use of a treatment plan.
- Complete an appointment card.
- Complete a daily schedule.
- Describe a call list.
- Explain advanced-function appointment scheduling.

SHORT-ANSWER OR FILL-IN QUESTIONS

1. List the information that should be entered in the appointment book when an appointment is made.

_____

_____

_____

_____

_____

_____

2. Explain how appointment scheduling in an advanced-function dental practice differs from scheduling in a traditional dental practice.

_____

_____

_____

_____

_____

_____

3. List six rules for efficient management of an appointment book.

1. _____

2. _____

3. _____

4. _____

5. _____

6. _____

MULTIPLE-CHOICE QUESTIONS

4. An outline of a dental appointment book is referred to as a:
   a. matrix.
   b. binder.
   c. context.
   d. scale down.

5. The objectives of good appointment book management include all *except* which of the following?
   a. Maximize productivity
   b. Reduce staff tension
   c. Maintain concern for patient needs
   d. Allow for maximum down time

6. Prime time in reference to appointment management refers to:
   a. the time during which the doctor wants to perform the most expensive type of dental treatment.
   b. the time most frequently requested by patients.
   c. the first 2 hours of the daily schedule.
   d. mid-day appointment times.

7. Which of the following types of treatment is commonly dovetailed in an appointment schedule?
   a. Dental laminate preparation
   b. Oral prophylaxis
   c. Denture adjustment
   d. Crown preparation

8. Which time of the day is considered most appropriate to treat young children?
   a. Just before naptime
   b. Immediately after naptime
   c. Early morning
   d. Late in the day

9. When scheduling (an) appointment(s) for a patient to have a three-unit fixed bridge, what is the minimum number of appointments needed?
   a. One
   b. Two
   c. Three
   d. Four

10. Which of the following units of time is *not* a common increment found in a dental appointment system?
    a. 10 minutes
    b. 15 minutes
    c. 30 minutes

11. What is the minimum number of appointments needed for a pulpectomy?
    a. One
    b. Two
    c. Three
    d. Four
    e. Five

12. The dentist informs you that the patient will need two appointments to complete a cast-metal crown. These appointments will be to:
    a. prepare the tooth and try in the crown.
    b. prepare the tooth and take an impression.
    c. prepare the tooth and seat the crown.
    d. take diagnostic models and make a temporary or provisional crown.

13. The dentist informs you that the patient will need three appointments to complete a three-unit bridge. These appointments will likely be to:
    a. prepare the teeth, try in the bridge components, and seat the bridge.
    b. take diagnostic models, prepare the teeth, and seat the temporary or provisional crown.
    c. prepare the teeth, take the impressions, and try in the components.

SOFTWARE TUTORIAL

Using the EagleSoft software you previously installed, modify the appointment book to reflect the times that a provider will be out of the office.

Directions for blocking out unavailable appointment times for the matrix are printed below. They can also be found by selecting the F1 key on your keyboard to access *Help* topics, clicking on the *Index* tab, and scrolling down to the topic *Blocking Unavailable Appointment Times*.

Blocking Unavailable Appointment Times

To block out chairs during times when the provider(s) might be unavailable:
1. Highlight the slot on the appointment grid that you wish to block from scheduling appointments.
2. Select *Block* or right-click on the appointment and choose *Create Block*. The *Block Appointment* window is displayed.
3. Enter the length of duration for the block. Do so by keying in the ending time in the To field or by entering the number of time units contained within the desired block.
4. Select the check box next to Block all chairs if you would like this block to be applied to all dental office chairs.
5. Enter any notes for the block in the Description field.
6. Select *OK* to apply the appointment block. The blocked time is displayed in charcoal gray to indicate that the time is unavailable for appointments. (If you do not wish to save the block, select *Cancel* to return to the *OnSchedule* tool.)

Using the EagleSoft software and the concepts discussed in the chapter, make appointments for patients who are already patients of record.

79

Appointment Book Matrix

Blocking the Schedule for One-Time Occurrences

■ Open the scheduling tool (*OnSchedule*), go to the day that needs to be blocked, click on the time, and select the *Block* button on the menu toolbar. Schedule the following times to be blocked:
  a. Dumont Study Club all day on the 9th
  b. Von Trapp Study Club all day on the 14th
  c. Western District Dental Society meeting all afternoon on the 20th
  d. Public school holiday on the 27th

Schedule Appointments

■ Open the scheduler by selecting the *OnSchedule* button on the toolbar or clicking on the monitor on the desktop that shows the scheduler.
■ Double-click on the appointment slot where the new appointment begins. You can also right-click in the appointment slot and choose the *Schedule Appointment* command.
■ Choose a patient name from the *Select Patient* window by highlighting the patient name and selecting *Use*. If the patient has an existing treatment plan, you are prompted to use the service codes from the treatment plan. If the patient has any alerts, they appear here as well.
■ If you need to add any services that have not been previously proposed on the patient's tooth chart, click on the *Service* button (bottom left) and add the services that will be necessary. This will also record the treatment on the patient's chart.
■ Make appointments for the following patients as indicated:
  a. Beth Burke calls and needs to set up an appointment for a prophylaxis. Schedule her also for four bite-wing radiographs. During the examination it is found that Beth Burke will need to have 18MO and 20DO restored with composite. Be sure that you add these new findings to her clinical chart and schedule that appointment. She wants to have this done as soon as possible because she has just taken a job as a television newscaster and wants to have an aesthetic restoration. She prefers an appointment between 1 and 4 PM.
  b. Set up appointments for Audra Chavez for all the proposed treatments on her clinical chart. (This information was input as part of the Software Tutorial exercises in Chapter 7.)
  c. Karmen Little has moved back to town after being away for some college work. She was in an automobile accident and lost teeth no. 23 through 26. The doctor has proposed doing a fixed bridge from no. 22 through 26. The abutment teeth will be no. 22 and 26 with porcelain fused to metal (PFM) crowns, with the four incisors being PFM pontics. Please update the clinical chart, and then make the necessary appointments for the bridge. Karmen is teaching some classes at the local community college and prefers late afternoon appointments after 3 PM. However, she has faculty meetings on Mondays, so that day is not a possible day for an appointment.
  d. Dennis Malone calls for an appointment for his prophylaxis. He cannot come in on Mondays or Wednesdays. He would also like to schedule an appointment to do a bleaching for both arches.
  e. Glenn Davis has not been to the office for some time. Set up an appointment for an adult prophylaxis and a periapical radiograph of no. 12 and four bite-wing radiographs.
  f. Rachel Burke was in today and needs to schedule her next appointment for 12^{MOD}, and she has also decided to have an external bleaching in the near future. She is a patient of record.
  g. Vicki Davis has a chart, but no treatment has been rendered. Today she had a prophylaxis, and the following teeth need to be charted on her tooth chart:

    No. 1 and 16 need to be removed.
    No. 4 has a MOD amalgam.
    No. 8 has decay on the mesial and needs to have a composite placed.

    She also needs to have an appointment for a periodontal maintenance procedure, deep scaling. Make the necessary appointments for this patient.
  h. Set up appointments for Catherine Gordon for all of the proposed treatment on her clinical chart. (This information was input as part of the *Software Tutorial* exercises in Chapter 7.)
  i. Set up appointments for Edward Raymond for all of the proposed treatment on his clinical chart. (This information was input as part of the *Software Tutorial* exercises in Chapter 7.)
■ Once these appointments have been entered, continue as though time has passed, make entries for each patient as though treatment has been completed, and produce walkout statements for each patient. The following patients were listed above for the treatment and have appointments in the near future, and treatment has been as follows:
  a. Beth Burke for a prophylaxis and four bitewing radiographs and the second appointment for 18MO and 20DO composite

Chapter **11** **Appointment Management Systems**

Copyright © 2011 by Mosby, Inc., an affiliate of Elsevier Inc. All rights reserved.

b. Audra Chavez for treatment on her clinical chart
c. Karmen Little for bridge preparation; abutment teeth: no. 22 and 26 with PFM crowns, with the four incisors being PFM pontics
d. Dennis Malone for a prophylaxis
e. Glenn Davis for an adult prophylaxis, a periapical radiograph of no. 12, and four bitewing radiographs
f. Rachel Burke for 12^{MOD} and an external bleaching
g. Vicki Davis for a prophylaxis, extraction of no. 1 and 16 and placement of a no. 8 mesial composite; also a periodontal maintenance procedure and deep scaling

CRITICAL THINKING ACTIVITIES

1. Explain why it is so important to consider the doctor's body clock when scheduling appointments. What could be the consequences of scheduling a complex procedure during a time when the doctor would not be at peak performance?

2. Consider an office with which you have been associated and identify problems that have occurred in scheduling that resulted in decreased productivity. How could some of these problems be resolved?

12 Recall Systems

A recall or recare system notifies patients of the timing of routine dental care. Some practitioners have adopted the term *recare* rather than recall, sensing that it suggests a more caring approach. Whether *recall* or *recare* is used as the term in the office, this system is an integral part of every modern dental practice and is essential to both the patient and the dentist. A recall-recare system is the lifeline of the practice. It helps to achieve one of the primary objectives of dentistry—helping patients maintain good oral health for a lifetime. The administrative assistant plays an integral role in maintaining this vitally important system in the practice. After reviewing the material in the textbook chapter, complete the activities in this workbook chapter to ensure that you have a thorough understanding of the recall-recare system used in the dental practice.

LEARNING OUTCOMES

On completion of text and workbook chapters, the student should be able to do the following:
- Define key terms.
- Explain the purpose of a recall or recare system.
- Describe motivational techniques to promote a recall or recare system.
- Identify different types of recall or recare systems.
- Develop a recall or recare system.

SHORT-ANSWER OR FILL-IN QUESTIONS

1. Describe the concept of a recall-recare system.

   _____

   _____

   _____

   _____

   _____

2. List six of the primary reasons that a patient would be placed on a recall-recare system.

   1. _____

   2. _____

   3. _____

   4. _____

   5. _____

   6. _____

3. Describe four systems of recall or recare.

1. _____

_____

2. _____

_____

3. _____

_____

4. _____

_____

4. Why is a recall system so important to a dental practice?

_____

_____

_____

5. Explain the advantages and disadvantages of each of the following types of systems.

Advanced Appointment System

_____

_____

_____

_____

_____

_____

Telephone Recall or Recare System

_____

_____

_____

_____

_____

_____

Mail Recall or Recare System

_____

_____

_____

_____

_____

_____

E-Mail and Text-Messaging Recall or Recare System

_____

_____

_____

_____

_____

_____

6. How has the computer made recall-recare an easier system to manage?

_____

_____

_____

7. What makes a recall-recare system function effectively?

_____

_____

_____

8. Which of the following statements is *not* true about a recall system?
   a. It is the lifeline of the dental practice.
   b. It is used solely for preventive recall.
   c. It can be used for follow-up endodontic treatment.
   d. It can be used to determine a child's eruption pattern.

9. The business assistant has failed to maintain the recall system for the past 4 months. Which of the following is likely to occur?
   a. Evidence of decreased productivity may occur.
   b. Patients will not mind.
   c. There will be more time to work on incomplete projects.

10. Which of the following is the *best* suggestion for a successful recall system?
    a. Using the telephone
    b. Using the mail
    c. Using e-mail
    d. Communication

11. Which of the recall systems takes the least amount of time and motion?
    a. Telephone
    b. Mail
    c. Advanced
    d. E-mail

12. To avoid potential litigation during a recall system's purge, the administrative assistant should:
    a. send a recall notice.
    b. send a letter informing the patient of recall record removal.
    c. phone the patient as soon as possible.
    d. ignore it because it is not an official record in the clinical chart.

SOFTWARE TUTORIAL

To understand how recall works in a dental software system, place the following patients on recall as listed:

Patient	Recall Time Frame
Beth Burke	4 months
Audra Chavez	6 months
Dennis Malone	6 months
Glenn Davis	4 months
Rachel Burke	6 months
Vicki Davis	3 months
Catherine Gordon	6 months
Edward Raymond	6 months

To do this, go to the *Person* window by selecting the *Person* button on the toolbar. Select the specific patient and go to the *Preference* button on the right side of the window. Enter the preferred recall frequency and save the information.

Note that patients Chavez, Malone, Burke, Gordon, and Raymond already have recall time frames set up. Verify the information and make any changes if necessary.

1. The business office manager is too busy to manage the recall system and fails to send recall notices to patients for the past 6 months. What impact does this have on the practice? What should be done about the management of this system?

2. How can you ensure that the office is using the most successful type of recall system available?

13 Inventory Systems and Supply Ordering

Making a dental office run smoothly can be a challenging experience in each area of the office. However, when a staff member reaches for a needed item and finds that it is not there, productivity and profitability can be diminished, whether it is the hygienist who reaches for a fluoride rinse and there is none available or the clinical assistant who suddenly realizes that there is no more of a specific dental cement. An effective inventory control system is invaluable, and it does not have to be complicated. Review the information in this chapter to learn about a variety of factors that can help to make the dental office become more organized in inventory control, and then complete the questions in this chapter of the workbook to ensure your understanding of the material.

LEARNING OUTCOMES

- Define key terms.
- Identify three types of dental supplies.
- Explain various types of inventory systems.
- Establish an inventory system.
- Explain factors determining supply quantity.
- Describe a technique for receiving supplies.
- Describe a computerized ordering system.
- Identify common supply forms.
- Explain the storage of hazardous materials.

SHORT-ANSWER OR FILL-IN QUESTIONS

1. List the information that is found on a material safety data sheet (MSDS).

   _____

   _____

   _____

   _____

2. Make a master supply list of 25 common expendable dental supplies and indicate the maximum and minimum levels based on the factors that determine supply amounts discussed in this chapter. Identify the manufacturer and, if possible, the most cost-effective supplier of these products in your area. You may want to visit a web site for suppliers listed in the chapter.

   1. _____

   2. _____

   3. _____

   4. _____

   5. _____

6. _____

7. _____

8. _____

9. _____

10. _____

11. _____

12. _____

13. _____

14. _____

15. _____

16. _____

17. _____

18. _____

19. _____

20. _____

21. _____

22. _____

23. _____

24. _____

25. _____

3. The items below were purchased as capital equipment. Fill out a card or enter into a database the following information:
   - A Delta Q 10-in. sterilizer was purchased and delivered today. The manufacturer is Pelton & Crane. It was purchased from Apex Dental Supply for $5173.90. The item code was 5531017, model number PC 182-4/84923. It has a warranty of 6 months from today.

_____

_____

_____

_____

_____

- A Nutorque Electric System programmable electric handpiece was delivered today. The manufacturer is StarDental, and it was purchased from Henry Schein Dental Supply. The item code is 8080884, and the model number is 8477. The cost was $2899.99 with a warranty for 1 year from today.

_____

_____

_____

_____

_____

4. List five questions that should be considered in an evaluation of the inventory system used in the office.

1. _____

2. _____

3. _____

4. _____

5. _____

5. List and explain the factors that aid in determining the minimum and maximum amounts of an item to be in inventory stock.

_____

_____

_____

_____

_____

_____

_____

_____

_____

_____

MATCHING

6. Select the definition from Column B that best defines the term in Column A.

Column A

_____ Back-order memo

_____ Capital supplies

_____ Credit memo

_____ Invoice

_____ MSDS

_____ Nonexpendable supplies

_____ Packing slip

_____ Purchase order

_____ Statement

_____ Expendable supplies

Column B

a. An enumeration of the items included in an order; it does not include the cost per item

b. A request for payment submitted by the dental supplier

c. A standardized form for ordering supplies

d. Large, costly items that are seldom replaced

e. Single-use items

f. A list of the contents of a package, the price of each item enclosed, and the total charge

g. A form supplied by the manufacturer that provides information about a hazardous material; these forms are required by the U.S. government

h. A form indicating that the dentist's account has been adjusted for the cost of a returned item

i. A form accompanying an order that notifies the purchaser that an item ordered is not currently in stock at the supply house and will be sent at a later date

j. Reusable items that do not constitute a major expense

MULTIPLE-CHOICE QUESTIONS

7. Which of the following information is *not* needed on a capital equipment inventory record?
   a. Date of purchase
   b. Manufacturer
   c. Serial number
   d. Dental sales person

8. Which of the following factors aids in determining the amount of a dental supply to order at one time?
   a. Rate of use
   b. Shelf life
   c. Amount of capital outlay
   d. Amount of storage
   e. All of the above

9. Which of the following items is a capital item?
   a. Contra angle
   b. Inkjet refill
   c. Computer
   d. Anesthetic syringe

10. Which of the following is an expendable item?
   a. Patient napkin
   b. Anesthetic syringe
   c. Spoon excavator
   d. Napkin chain

11. Which of the following is a nonexpendable item?
   a. Patient napkin
   b. Anesthetic syringe
   c. Inkjet refill
   d. Computer paper

There appears to be a trend in the office that is causing the clinical assistants to run out of supplies in the treatment rooms during the middle of the day's procedures. This issue was brought up in a staff meeting. What might the causes be, and how could this situation be resolved?

14 Dental Insurance

Although the United States has been faced with major changes in insurance coverage for patients, its emergence and growth have provided access to care for people who had never considered routine dental treatment. Dental insurance is a major part of the dental business office and requires that the administrative assistant be well aware of the importance of following standard protocols in completing the forms necessary to obtain reimbursement for the dentist's services rendered. It is impossible to bring to the reader the latest version of *Current Dental Terminology* references because they change regularly; so it will benefit the student to have access to the most current documents in the office or classroom or obtain them from the web site of the American Dental Association (www.ada.org).

Review the materials in this chapter, answer the questions, and then complete the insurance claim forms using the EagleSoft software that accompanies this book. If you are currently working in a dental office, you may want to use the actual software and an insurance claim that needs to be processed to ensure your understanding of this chapter.

LEARNING OUTCOMES

On completion of text and workbook chapters, the student should be able to do the following:
- Define key terms.
- Identify the four parties affected by dental benefit plans.
- Differentiate among the different dental plan models.
- Use the current American Dental Association (ADA) *Code on Dental Procedures and Nomenclature and the Code of Dental Terminology (CDT) manual.*
- Complete an ADA form.
- Submit Medicaid dental benefit claims.
- Apply the rules for coordination of benefits.
- Explain common dental benefit and claims terminology.

SHORT-ANSWER OR FILL-IN QUESTIONS

1. List and explain the four parties involved in dental insurance delivery.

    1. _____

        _____

    2. _____

        _____

    3. _____

        _____

    4. _____

        _____

2. How does the Health Insurance Portability and Accountability Act (HIPAA) affect dental healthcare providers who transmit claim forms electronically?

_____

_____

_____

3. What is a National Provider Identifier (NPI)?

_____

_____

_____

4. Describe coordination of benefits (COB) as it applies to a dental plan.

_____

_____

_____

_____

5. Explain and list the categories of codes that are published in the CDT. To ensure that you have the most current codes, consult the latest edition or version of the CDT.

_____

_____

_____

_____

_____

_____

_____

_____

_____

_____

_____

_____

MATCHING EXERCISES

6. Match the term in Column A with the definition in Column B.

Column A	Column B
_____ Assignment of benefits	a. Fee-for-service dental benefits program in which payment of benefits is based on reasonable and customary fee criteria
_____ Capitation	b. A request form used for payment or predetermination for patients covered by a dental benefits program
_____ Claim form	c. The employee or participant who is certified by the company or organization (group) providing the dental program as eligible to receive benefit coverage
_____ Co-payment	d. A dental benefits program in which payment for covered benefits is based on a combination of usual, customary, and reasonable fees criteria
_____ CDT	e. Benefits system in which a dentist contracts with the program to provide all or most of the dental services covered under the program in return for a fixed monthly payment per covered person
_____ Dependent	f. A method of determining the primary carrier for dependent children who are covered by more than one dental plan using the primary payer as the parent with the earlier date of birth by month and day, without regard to the year of birth
_____ Subscriber	g. Federal act that allows a person to maintain insurance coverage temporarily, even if he or she loses the job through which coverage was obtained
_____ COBRA	h. Method of determining the primary carrier for dependent children who are covered by more than one dental plan using the father as the primary payer
_____ Birthday rule	i. Individuals, such as a spouse and children, who are legally and contractually eligible for benefits under a subscriber's benefit package
_____ Gender rule	j. The amount or percentage of the dentist's fee that the patient is obligated to pay
_____ UCR plan	k. Authorization by the enrollee or patient for the dental benefits carrier to make payment for covered services directly to the treating dentist
_____ R and C plan	l. A reference manual developed by the ADA that includes the Code on Dental Procedures and Nomenclature and other instructional tools for reporting dental services to dental benefits plans and administrators

MULTIPLE-CHOICE QUESTIONS

7. A dental benefits program in which enrollees can receive benefits only when services are provided by dentists who have signed an agreement with the benefit plan to provide treatment to eligible patients is referred to as a:
   a. closed panel system.
   b. UCR system.
   c. R and C system.
   d. COBRA system.

8. The fee most often charged by the dentist or that is adjusted in consideration of the nature and severity of the condition treated and any medical or dental complications or unusual circumstances that may affect treatment is referred to as the:
   a. usual fee.
   b. customary fee.
   c. reasonable fee.

97

9. The fee that a dentist most frequently charges for a given dental service is the:
   a. usual fee.
   b. customary fee.
   c. reasonable fee.

10. Which of the following will *not* be accepted on a claim form by an insurance company?
    a. Primary subscriber
    b. Child's nickname
    c. Date of birth
    d. Fee for service

11. An insurance company requests verification of a patient's birth date and complete name. A copy of the patient's entire record is sent to the company, including the health history indicating evidence of HIV. This action may be considered:
    a. fraud.
    b. violation of confidentiality.
    c. assault and battery.
    d. defamation of character.

12. When using the ADA *Code on Dental Procedures and Nomenclature* to complete an insurance claim form, which of the following codes is *not* defined accurately?
    a. The letter "D" throughout the series and identifying all procedures as being dental
    b. The second digit denoting the category of service
    c. The third designating the class of a specific procedure
    d. The fourth digit provided for expansion of the code

13. A patient has insurance coverage from July 1 of last year until June 30 of this year, after which time the patient will no longer receive this benefit. The patient had a maximum benefit coverage of $1200. For the year and to date the patient had used only $450 of the benefit. Toward the end of June it is determined that the patient needed to have two laminates. The work cannot be completed before July 1. The patient is informed of the fee for the bridge. The patient insists that because she has more than $700 unused balance from her insurance that the doctor should change the date of the service to ensure that the fee will be covered by the insurance. To do this the dentist will be committing:
    a. abandonment.
    b. breach of contract.
    c. fraud.
    d. negligence.

14. The term *subscriber* (or *policyholder*) used in insurance management refers to the
    a. dentist.
    b. employer.
    c. male spouse.
    d. the employee who represents the family unit in relation to the prepayment plan.

15. Which of the following data is *not* required on an insurance claim form?
    a. Patient name
    b. Subscriber's name
    c. Dentist identification number or social security number
    d. Dentist's birth date

16. A dependent on an insurance claim form refers to the
    a. spouse or children.
    b. dentist.
    c. employee.

SOFTWARE TUTORIAL

With software systems the insurance form is frequently created as part of the patient "workout" or posting of charges. To practice insurance charges within the EagleSoft software system, perform the following steps:

1. Make an appointment for patient Lori Taylor on today's date (at a time later than the current time). By selecting the *Service* button, add that Lori is coming in for an adult prophylaxis, four bitewing x-rays, and an examination.
2. Save and close the appointment.
3. The next step, the posting of charges, has many options based on the office that is using the software. For this exercise, reopen the appointment and click on the *Fast Walkout* button.
4. The first window will show what services are going to be charged to the patient. Click *Process*.
5. The second window allows for the entry of payments made during the appointment. For now leave these blank, and click *OK*.
6. The third window is the insurance form. Look at the formatting for different forms using the *Insurance Form* drop-down field. You will notice that both blank and regular versions of most forms are available. The blank version just allows the option to print the form. Having this window allows the assistant to insert notes and answer any questions applicable to the patient's visit. The form can then be set to print later, print immediately, or be sent electronically.
7. When you click the *OK* button, the charges are entered, the insurance form is completed, and the patient's tooth chart is updated.

CRITICAL THINKING ACTIVITY

Explain how the administrative assistant determines the primary carrier when a patient has COB.

15 Financial Systems: Accounts Receivable

As discussed in various areas of the textbook, dentistry is a business as well as a health profession. In this chapter the reader will understand that sound business practices must be integrated into the management of the dental office to maintain a steady cash flow and a solvent practice. Emphasis in this chapter is on accounts receivable, which includes all production; data are entered for treatment rendered, payments received, and account adjustments made, and new balances are calculated. Review the chapter and then proceed to complete the activities in this chapter of the workbook to ensure that you have a thorough understanding of common bookkeeping and business procedures used in a modern dental practice.

LEARNING OUTCOMES

On completion of text and workbook chapters, the student should be able to do the following:
- Define key terms.
- Define *bookkeeping*.
- Define *accounting*.
- Explain basic mathematical procedures.
- Describe common bookkeeping systems in dentistry.
- Explain the function of a computerized accounts receivable program.
- Explain the production of patient statements.
- Identify common payment and credit policies.
- Describe the various laws affecting credit policies and collection procedures.
- Describe the "red flags" rule.
- Identify common problsems in maintaining a credit policy.
- Identify the functions of a credit bureau.
- Explain the function of a collection agency.
- Compose collection letters.

SHORT-ANSWER OR FILL-IN QUESTIONS

1. Explain how a patient statement is generated and when these statements should be sent to patients. At what other time could a patient receive a statement?

   _____

   _____

   _____

2. List the components of a well-defined credit policy for the office.

   _____

   _____

   _____

   _____

   _____

3. Explain how identity theft could occur in a dental office.

_____

_____

_____

4. List 10 rules that should be followed when using the telephone for collections.

1. _____

2. _____

3. _____

4. _____

5. _____

6. _____

7. _____

8. _____

9. _____

10. _____

5. List four suggestions for selecting an ethical and reliable collection agency.

1. _____

2. _____

3. _____

4. _____

6. What information should be given to a collection agency to enable the company's representatives to collect an account?

_____

_____

_____

_____

_____

_____

_____

7. What is the function of a credit bureau?

_____

_____

_____

8. Explain six rules that should be followed in composing an effective collection letter.

1. _____

2. _____

3. _____

4. _____

5. _____

6. _____

9. When an account is turned over to a collection agency, what should be the role of the dental office staff?

_____

_____

_____

_____

_____

MATCHING EXERCISE

10. Match the term in Column A with the definition in Column B.

Column A	Column B
_____ Accounting	a. A form given to the payer (patient) that acknowledges payment on an account
_____ Accounts payable	b. A document that informs patients of their financial status with the dentist; it indicates the charges, payments, and balances on an account for the month just concluded
_____ Accounts receivable	c. All the dentist's financial obligations or money that the dentist owes (outgoing money)
_____ Adjustment	d. An organization that reports specific information about a person's previous payment habits on deferred payment plans
_____ Balance	e. An amount owed to the dentist for services rendered
_____ Bookkeeping	f. An institution or business that sends a bill to a person, agrees to an installment payment plan, accepts insurance payments, or arranges for a loan for payment
_____ Credit balance	g. An amount owed to the patient for services for which the dentist has been paid in advance but that have not yet been performed
_____ Credit bureau	h. The amount on an account, whether credit or debit, before activity was posted to the account
_____ Creditor	i. A check returned unpaid to the payee because insufficient funds were available in the payer's account
_____ Debit balance	j. The credit or debit amount on an account
_____ NSF check	k. The process of recording of financial transactions
_____ Previous balance	l. Alteration of an account balance as a result of a courtesy discount, the return of a nonsufficient funds check, or a payment
_____ Receipt	m. A category that includes all production; data are entered for treatment rendered and payments received, and new balances are calculated
_____ Statement	n. The recording, classifying, and summarizing of financial and business records, generally the task of the accountant

MULTIPLE-CHOICE QUESTIONS

11. When searching for a patient record in financial software, which of the following commands might likely be used?
    a. Add
    b. Find
    c. Del
    d. Enter

12. Which of the following commands would you use in computer software when you wish to leave the screen?
    a. Edit
    b. Enter
    c. Esc
    d. File

13. Which of the following commands would you use in a computer software system to enter data or create a new patient record?
    a. Add
    b. Edit
    c. Esc
    d. File

Chapter **15** **Financial Systems: Accounts Receivable**

14. Which of the following commands would you use in a computer software system to find a patient, an account, or other data?
    a. Edit
    b. File
    c. Locate
    d. Post

15. Which of the following commands would you use in a computer software system to eliminate part or all of the data entry?
    a. Edit
    b. Del
    c. Esc
    d. File

SOFTWARE TUTORIAL

Use the EagleSoft software system to make entries for each of the patients and the activities listed below. Please review the technique for using the CD-ROM before making the entries.

In Chapters 11 and 14, charges were entered for several patients. In addition, there were patients of record already in the system with account balances. Make entries for accounts receivable, which will be from checks received directly from the patient or from insurance payments received in the mail.

To enter payments for specific patients, go to the account window for the patient by clicking on the *Account* button on the toolbar at the top or the drawer on the office front desk window (*Practice Management* mode). Then select the correct patient account. Select *Account Payment* to enter the payment into the patient record. To enter insurance payments, go to the *Claim* button on the front desk toolbar; highlight the correct claim and select the *Make Payment* button.

Process payments for the following patients, for whom appointments and treatments were scheduled and completed in Chapter 11:

- Personal check (no. 1254) received from John Abbott for $425.00
- Personal check (no. 567) from Beth Burke for $200.00
- Credit card payment (Visa) from Rachael Burke for $178.20

To practice making additional payment entries, go to the appointment book and make an appointment for a patient. Click on *Fast Walkout* and enter the appropriate charges. You will then be able to post payments.

CRITICAL THINKING ACTIVITY

Why is it so important to place a responsible person in charge of the accounts receivable system even if you use a computer software system?

Chapter **15**   **Financial Systems: Accounts Receivable**

16 Other Financial Systems

All dental practices, regardless of size, have financial matters that need to be addressed by either internal or external accounting staff. The administrative assistant can expect to perform many tasks in addition to the accounts receivable activities discussed in the previous chapter. These tasks might include receiving and organizing statements, paying for materials and supplies, processing payroll or tax forms, recording and analyzing expenses, and other responsibilities.

In a group practice or a larger organization, the administrative assistant may collect the data for these activities and support accounting personnel in the preparation of financial documents, or he or she may be responsible for entering data in a software package such as QuickBooks. However, many offices still perform these tasks manually, and the administrative assistant must have a basic understanding of the financial systems involved and be able to provide the necessary data for management of the financial system. Review the materials in the corresponding textbook chapter, and then complete the questions and activities in this workbook chapter to ensure that you have a thorough understanding of other financial systems used in the dental practice.

LEARNING OUTCOMES

On completion of the text and workbook chapters, the student should be able to do the following:
- Define key terms.
- Explain the function of a budget.
- Explain the use of electronic banking.
- Describe the steps in accessing an online bank account.
- Identify the parts of a check.
- Explain the use of financial management software.
- Prepare a check and determine the correct balance on a checkbook register.
- Identify various types of checks.
- Prepare checks for deposit with correct endorsements and complete a deposit slip.
- Reconcile a bank statement.
- Explain the purpose of a monthly expense sheet.
- Explain the purpose of a yearly summary.
- Identify the purpose of payroll records.
- Explain the purpose of the employee's earnings record.
- Calculate gross and net wages.
- Explain how withheld income tax and Social Security taxes are deposited.
- Explain how federal unemployment taxes are deposited.
- Describe how to complete a Form W-2.
- Explain the importance of retaining payroll records.
- Explain the use of an automated payroll system.
- Use the Internet as a resource for financial forms and instructions.

1. Describe the procedures for reconciling a bank statement.

_____

_____

_____

_____

_____

_____

2. List eight advantages to using financial software, such as QuickBooks®.

1. _____

2. _____

3. _____

4. _____

5. _____

6. _____

7. _____

8. _____

3. Identify five important factors to remember when using an ATM.

1. _____

2. _____

3. _____

4. _____

5. _____

4. Identify the information that should be included in the employee's earnings record, which is used for various state and federal reports.

_____

_____

_____

_____

_____

_____

_____

5. Explain the difference between gross and net wages.

_____

_____

6. What is the purpose of Form 941, and when is the form prepared?

_____

_____

_____

_____

_____

_____

_____

_____

_____

7. What information is included on Form W-2?

_____

_____

_____

_____

_____

_____

_____

8. Explain the importance of payroll and tax record retention.

_____

_____

_____

_____

_____

MULTIPLE-CHOICE QUESTIONS

9. Which of the following is *not* a rule for entering data on financial records?
   a. Decimal points are not necessary.
   b. Make a backup of a computer file.
   c. Always use ink when making manual entries.
   d. Check mathematic computations.

10. A personal check that has a guarantee that the funds have been set aside by the bank for payment of the check is a
    a. cashier's check.
    b. certified check.
    c. money order.
    d. traveler's check.

11. A check that a bank draws on its funds in another bank is a bank draft.
    a. True
    b. False

12. Reconciliation of the bank balance is the balancing of the bank statement with the check stub-check register balance.
    a. True
    b. False

13. The petty cash fund requires less control than the checking account.
    a. True
    b. False

14. A check that is preprinted in various denominations is referred to as a
    a. money order.
    b. certified check.
    c. traveler's check.
    d. voucher check.

15. The petty cash fund should always maintain $100.00. Today the balance remaining in this fund is $17.39. For which amount should a check be written to maintain the petty cash fund?
    a. $100.00
    b. $17.39
    c. $82.61
    d. $28.61

16. If a patient used a debit card, which of the following is *not* true?
    a. It is actually an electronic check.
    b. The funds may be withdrawn directly from bank account.
    c. The fund may be withdrawn from a remaining balance on a prepaid debit card.
    d. It is the same as a credit card.

17. An endorsement that indicates *for deposit only* is a/an
    a. blank endorsement.
    b. endorsement in full.
    c. restrictive endorsement.

18. Checks not yet returned to the bank on a bank statement are
    a. NSF checks.
    b. outstanding checks.
    c. expired checks.
    d. returned checks.

19. The amount of money withheld from an employee's pay check depends on
    a. the number of exemptions indicated on Form W-4.
    b. the number of exemptions indicated on Form W-2.
    c. the marital status of the employee.
    d. the amount of the gross pay.

20. A wage and tax statement for a calendar year must be provided for each employee no later than
    a. December 31 of the calendar year of employment.
    b. January 31 of the following year.
    c. April 15 of the following year.
    d. March 15 of the following year.

21. Identify the parts of the check as shown in the illustration.

1. _____

2. _____

3. _____

4. _____

5. _____

6. _____

7. _____

8. _____

9. _____

10. _____

11. _____

MATCHING EXERCISE

22. Match the term in Column A with the definition in Column B.

Column A	Column B
_____ ABA	a. The total amount of earnings after deductions
_____ ATM	b. The amount of money withheld for federal and state taxes
_____ Bank deposit	c. The amount of money spent to operate a business or practice
_____ Bank draft	d. A wage and tax statement for a calendar year must be provided for each employee no later than January 31 of the following year
_____ Bank statement	e. A check for which a guarantee exists that funds have been set aside to cover the amount of the check
_____ Budget	f. The federal form used to determine the status of each employee for income tax deductions from wages
_____ Cashier's check	g. A law that requires deductions for social security and Medicare taxes

_____	Certified check	h. A printed document from the bank showing the balance of the account at the beginning of the month, deposits made during the month, checks drawn against the account, corrections or charges against the account, and the bank balance at the end of the month
_____	Checks	i. The signature or stamp of the payee
_____	Form W-4	j. A financial plan of operation for a given period, usually 1 year
_____	Employer identification number	k. The total amount of earnings before deductions
_____	Endorsement	l. A means of ordering the bank to pay cash from a bank customer's account
_____	Expenditures	m. Represents the accumulation of money received for a single day or possibly a longer period
_____	FICA	n. The bank's own order to make payment out of the bank's funds
_____	Form SS-4	o. A small amount of cash kept on hand in the office to pay for small expenses
_____	Gross wages	p. A nine-digit number assigned to sole proprietors or corporations for filing and reporting payroll information
_____	Money order	q. A means of transferring money without using cash or a personal check
_____	Net pay	r. A national organization of banks and holding companies of all sizes that deals with issues of importance to national institutions
_____	Petty cash	s. The application form used to obtain an employer identification number
_____	Revenue	t. A check that provides a detachable stub, which can be used as an accounting record for itemizing payment of invoices or any type of itemization the payer would like as a reference
_____	Traveler's check	u. A payment device purchased through a bank or other agency that serves as cash for a person who is away from home
_____	Voucher check	v. A check drawn by the cashier of one bank on another bank in which the first bank has available funds on deposit or credit
_____	Form W-2	w. A computer workstation that electronically prompts the user through most routine banking activities
_____	Withholding	x. The amount of income received by a business or practice

PRACTICAL ACTIVITIES

Copy and use the following blank check and deposit forms to complete the following exercises.

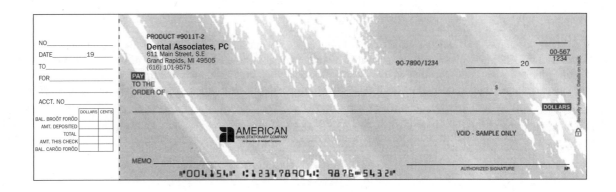

RESERVED FOR BANK USE

PLEASE LIST EACH CHECK SEPARATELY	DOLLARS	CENTS
CURRENCY		
SILVER		
Checks		
TOTAL		
LESS CASH RETURNED		
TOTAL DEPOSIT		

PLEASE ENDORSE ALL CHECKS AND DRAFTS
Deposited for Account of

_____

_____

ADDRESS _____

DATE _____

ACCOUNT NUMBER

23. Using sample checks and deposit slips, write the proper information on the check stubs and checks for Dental Associates, PC. The corporate name is imprinted on the checks, and the bank's identification number and corporate account number have been encoded on the checks for "reading" by the bank's electronic equipment. Prepare the check stubs, checks, and deposit slips for the following transactions, using the current year for the date on each:

May 1, 20–
The balance in the checking account is $75,769.52. Record this balance (balance brought forward).

May 2, 20–
Number the first check 114. Make it payable to the ADA for a seminar on infection control update in the amount of $175.00.

May 4, 20–
Deposit $10,719.62 in the bank.

May 5, 20–
Issue check no. 115 for $27,325.60, payable to ADP Payroll Services for the biweekly payroll.

May 8, 20–
Deposit $2385.81 in the bank.

May 10, 20–
Issue check no. 116 for $4416.85, payable to John T. Snyder & Sons, for painting the office.

May 11, 20–
Deposit $5667.16 in the bank.

May 14, 20–
Issue check no. 117 for $60.50, payable to the Magazine Clearinghouse, for three magazine subscriptions for the office.

May 17, 20–
Deposit $10,657.20 in the bank.

May 19, 20–
Issue check no. 118 for $27,929.60, payable to ADP Payroll Services, for the biweekly payroll.

May 22, 20–
Issue check no. 119 for $2500.00, payable to Health Science Dental Supply Co., as the balance of payment on a dental unit.

May 24, 20–
Deposit $8225.50 in the bank.

May 24, 20–
Issue check no. 120 for $370.84, payable to Computer Depot, for a new DVD player.

May 26, 20–
Deposit $18,308.20 in the bank.

May 25, 20—
Issue check no. 121 to American City Bank for $4890.00 to pay the mortgage.

May 26, 20–
Issue check no. 122 for $350.80, payable to Uniforms Unlimited.

May 28, 20–
Issue check no. 123 for $950.00, payable to Meyer Dental Co., for dental supplies.

May 28, 20–
Issue check no. 124 for $71.60, payable to "Cash," to replenish the petty cash fund.

May 29, 20–
Deposit $13,179.40 in the bank.

May 29, 20–
Issue check no. 125 for $287.55, payable to Johnson Printing Co., for stationery and envelopes.

May 31, 20–
Deposit $3924.16 in the bank.

24. Use the following information to complete a deposit slip. Deposit to the account of Dental Associates, PC; the account number is 9876-5432.
   a. Calculate the total of the following deposit:

   Currency: $900.00
   Silver: $0.75
   Checks: ABA numbers 12-456, 03-471, 21-689, 31-82, 79-43, 66-101, with respective amounts of $350.00, $340.75, $475.00, $45.80, $180.90, and $920.10
   Cash returned: None

   b. Calculate the total of the following deposit:

   Currency: $264.00
   Silver: $0.85
   Money order: $60.00;
   Checks: ABA numbers 14-957, 56-123, 43-210, 89-567, 44-056, with respective amounts of $460.00, $390.00, $189.59, $85.00, $190.00
   Cash returned: $50.00

25. On July 25 you received the bank statement for parts of the months of June and July with a balance of $47,790.47. After examining the transactions for the months, you note that a deposit for $500.00 made on July 20 does not appear on the bank's statement. Also, checks no. 2008 ($1100.00), no. 2014 ($256.00), and no. 2025 ($75.00) have not cleared the bank. Check no. 2005, incorrectly recorded on the check stubs as $67.20, should have been $76.20. The checkbook balance at this time is $46,859.47. Reconcile the bank statement and checkbook to the adjusted balance.

26. Perform the following computations:
   a. Determine the weekly gross wages for the following four employees. Forty hours is the regular workweek. Overtime is paid at one and a half times the regular rate of pay for any hours over 40 during the week.
      (1) Mario Garcia: $1182.50 weekly; married, two exemptions

(2) Mary O'Brian: 41 hours, $19.50 per hour; married, zero exemptions

(3) Keith Sams: 48 hours, $26.50 per hour; married, three exemptions

(4) Betty Todd: 43.5 hours, $28.50 per hour; married, one exemption

b. Figure the weekly deductions for each of the employees in Part A using the following information:
   ■ Federal Insurance Contributions Act (FICA): 7.65%
   ■ Withholding tax: Current IRS withholding tables and a calculator are available at www.irs.gov.
   ■ Credit union: $50.00 for O'Brian and Todd and $100.00 for Garcia
   ■ Life insurance: $27.60 for each employee

   1. Mario Garcia

   2. Mary O'Brian

   3. Keith Sams

   4. Betty Todd

c. Determine the weekly net wages for each of the four employees.
   1. Mario Garcia

   2. Mary O'Brian

   3. Keith Sams

   4. Betty Todd

27. Assume that Carla Simmons has earned $106,200.00 by November 15, 2009. She earns $2310.00 weekly. (For 2009 FICA is calculated at 7.65%, which is split between Social Security at 6.2% on the first $106,800.00 earned in the year and Medicare at 1.45% on all earnings with no yearly cap.) How much of her weekly earnings will be taxable for FICA? What amount of FICA tax will she pay?

28. With the following information, complete the W-2 form (copy on p. 119 and also available at www.irs.gov) using the following employee information:

Name: Betty Todd
Address: 2035 East Maplewood, Grand Rapids, MI 49506
Social Security number: 833-43-7044
Employer: Dental Associates, PC, 611 Main Street, SE, Grand Rapids, MI 49502
Tax No.: 430038178
Total wages taxable for state, federal, and FICA: $62,240.00
Employee's deductions for the year:
- Federal income tax: $4056.00
- State income tax: $626.20
- FICA: $4761.00, of which $902.00 was for Medicare and remainder was for Social Security

Chapter **16** **Other Financial Systems**

22222	**a** Employee's social security number				
		OMB No. 1545-0008			

b Employer identification number (EIN)		**1** Wages, tips, other compensation	**2** Federal income tax withheld
c Employer's name, address, and ZIP code		**3** Social security wages	**4** Social security tax withheld
		5 Medicare wages and tips	**6** Medicare tax withheld
		7 Social security tips	**8** Allocated tips
d Control number		**9** Advance EIC payment	**10** Dependent care benefits
e Employee's first name and initial Last name Suff.		**11** Nonqualified plans	**12a** Code
		13 Statutory employee Retirement plan Third-party sick pay	**12b** Code
		14 Other	**12c** Code
			12d Code
f Employee's address and ZIP code			

15 State Employer's state ID number	**16** State wages, tips, etc.	**17** State income tax	**18** Local wages, tips, etc.	**19** Local income tax	**20** Locality name

Form **W-2** **Wage and Tax Statement**   **2009**   Department of the Treasury—Internal Revenue Service

Copy 1—For State, City, or Local Tax Department

Note: This is a copy of Form W-2 provided by the IRS for informational purposes only and is not intended to be filed. Official copies for filing should be obtained directly from the IRS.

CRITICAL THINKING ACTIVITIES

29. Why would a dentist be concerned about having the office manager bonded? What is involved in this process?

30. Think about the qualifications of the office manager or administrative assistant in relation to the financial systems used in the dental office. How could a background in business benefit the dentist owner of the practice? What issues might need to be resolved if the person in the administrative assistant's position had only a background in business and no dental education? How could these issues be resolved?

17 Infection Control Systems

An administrative assistant generally has no direct patient contact. However, this person must understand both the risks and management of occupational exposures to blood-borne pathogens. Although his or her primary duties are in the business office, the administrative assistant may be called on to perform a clinical task that could cause exposure to such a risk. The assigned job, therefore, does not make it impossible to contract a communicable disease. There is a great deal of information regarding infection control in this chapter. Review it thoroughly, and then complete the questions in this workbook to ensure that you can work safely in the business office of a dental practice.

LEARNING OUTCOMES

On completion of text and workbook chapters, the student should be able to do the following:
- Define key terms.
- Identify the importance to the administrative assistant of an understanding of disease transmission.
- Identify the routes of disease transmission.
- Describe basic infection control procedures.
- Identify the various regulatory agencies that impact the dental office.
- Identify the various records required by the Occupational Safety and Health Administration that must be maintained in the business office.
- Explain routine procedures that the administrative assistant might perform to maintain quality assurance in the office.

SHORT-ANSWER OR FILL-IN QUESTIONS

1. Why is it so important to have a copy of the *Guidelines for Infection Control in Dental Health Care Settings* in the dental office*?* What are the major components of this book?

_____

_____

_____

_____

_____

_____

2. Describe two types of infections.

1. _____

_____

2. _____

_____

3. Explain how infection can be transmitted.

_____

_____

_____

4. The doctor asks you to set up a health program for the staff to ensure that they are all current in the latest information. What should be included in the office's personnel policy as it relates to a health protection program for the staff?

_____

_____

_____

_____

_____

_____

_____

5. What are the goals of standard precautions in the workplace?

_____

_____

_____

6. List six records that should be maintained for each dental healthcare worker (DHCW).

1. _____

2. _____

3. _____

4. _____

5. _____

6. _____

7. List eight items that should be kept readily available for use in preventing or dealing with a hazardous spill.

    1. _____

    2. _____

    3. _____

    4. _____

    5. _____

    6. _____

    7. _____

    8. _____

8. List eight procedures commonly used to maintain asepsis and prevent cross contamination in the dental office.

    1. _____

    2. _____

    3. _____

    4. _____

    5. _____

    6. _____

    7. _____

    8. _____

9. Match the term in Column A with the definition in Column B.

Column A

_____ AIDS

_____ Antiseptic
_____ Autogenous infection

_____ Bioburden
_____ Blood-borne pathogens

_____ Centers for Disease Control and Prevention (CDC)
_____ Communicable disease
_____ Cross contamination

_____ DHCW

_____ Disinfection

_____ Environmental Protection Agency

_____ Hazardous waste

_____ Hepatitis B virus

_____ Infection
_____ Infectious waste

_____ Occupational Safety and Health Administration (OSHA)

_____ Personal protective equipment (PPE)
_____ Sepsis

_____ Sharp containers

_____ Sterilization

_____ Standard precautions

Column B

a. The process of rendering an item free of germs; commonly achieved by steam under pressure, dry heat, or chemical vapor

b. A pathologic state characterized by the presence of pathogens

c. A disease that may be transmitted directly or indirectly from one individual to another

d. Another name for AIDS

e. Self-produced infection; originating within the body

f. Materials identified as hazardous to human health; local, state, and federal regulations require special handling of such materials

g. A federal agency that regulates the use and disposal of hazardous materials

h. Any substance that interferes with the sterilization process

i. Organisms transmitted through blood or blood products that can cause infectious diseases

j. A dental professional who provides care to patients or has some contact with dental patients in the office

k. Invasion of body tissues by disease-producing microorganisms and the reaction of the tissues to these microorganisms or their toxins (or both)

l. A federal agency responsible for investigating the incidence of disease, monitoring diseases throughout the world, and conducting research directed toward controlling and preventing disease

m. The transfer of impurities, infection, or disease from one source to another

n. A federal agency that establishes guidelines and regulations for worker safety

o. The process of destroying some pathogenic microorganisms

p. The process used to maintain an aseptic field and to prevent cross contamination and cross infection between healthcare providers, between healthcare providers and patients, and between patients

q. Virus that causes a form of hepatitis B that is transmitted in contaminated serum in blood transfusions, in the passing of contaminated fluids, or by use of contaminated needles and instruments

r. Enclosed device from which an article cannot be retrieved

s. An antimicrobial agent that can be applied to a body surface, usually skin or raw mucosa, to try to prevent or minimize infection in the area of application

t. Materials used to protect the employee when occupational exposure is possible, such as disposable gloves, disposable surgical masks and gowns, laboratory coats and scrubs, and face shields or eye protection with side shields

u. A disease caused by a retrovirus known as the human immunodeficiency virus type 1 (HIV-1). A related but distinct retrovirus (HIV-2) has recently appeared in a limited number of patients in the United States.

v. Blood and blood products, contaminated sharps, pathologic wastes, and microbiologic waste

10. Infection control in the dental office is the responsibility of
    a. the dentist.
    b. the clinical dental assistant.
    c. the dental hygienist.
    d. the office manager.
    e. all dental staff.

11. Which of the following is an improper technique as it relates to infection control in the dental office?
    a. Storing instruments in sealed bags
    b. Placing patient records outside the treatment room
    c. Eating in the laboratory or other contaminated site
    d. Changing gloves for each patient

12. Which of the following is not a regulatory record that needs to be retained?
    a. Exposure determination form
    b. Employee training records
    c. Employee medical records
    d. FUTA

13. The role of the CDC is to enforce regulations set forth by OSHA to protect the health, safety, and welfare of the public and dental personnel.
    a. True
    b. False

14. Little concern should be given to patient records in the treatment room because microorganisms are not attracted to flat surfaces.
    a. True
    b. False

15. Who determines the hazards of a dental material?
    a. Employer
    b. Employee
    c. Manufacturer
    d. Dental distributor

16. The administrative assistant is immune from disease transmission because he or she does not have direct patient contact.
    a. True
    b. False

PRACTICAL ACTIVITY

Using the sample form provided on p. 126, complete an accident report for the following situation:

The clinical dental assistant, Rachel F. Thompson, experienced a needle puncture while Mr. Frank Oliver was being treated. The assistant's address is 4001 Kinect Drive, Cutlerville, MI 49545, SSN 000-00-2111, birth date 4/17/89. The accident occurred in Dr. Ashley Lake's office while the dentist was returning the syringe to the assistant at chair side, resulting in a needle poke to the middle finger of the left hand. The assistant's physician, Gerald Murphy, MD, was contacted for follow-up, but no hospitalization was necessary. The dentist is Ashley M. Lake (The address and other data can be obtained from Chapter 7.)

Bureau of Statistics
Supplementary Record of
Occupational Injuries and Illnesses

U.S. Department of Labor

This form is required by Public Law 91-596 and must be kept in the establishment for 5 years. Failure to maintain can result in the issuance of citations and assessment of penalties.	Case or File No.	Form approved O.M.B. No. 1220-0029

Employer

1. Name

2. Mail address *(No. and street, city or town, State, and zip code)*

3. Location, if different from mail address

Injured or Ill Employee

4. Name *(First, middle, and last)* — Social Security No.

5. Home address *(No. and street, city or town, State, and zip code)*

6. Age

7. Sex: *(Check one)* Male ☐ Female ☐

8. Occupation *(Enter regular job title*, not *the specific activity he was performing at the time of injury.)*

9. Department *(Enter name of department or division in which the injured person is regularly employed, even though he may have been temporarily working in another department at the time of injury.)*

The Accident or Exposure to Occupational Illness

If accident or exposure occurred on employer's premises, give address of plant or establishment in which it occurred. Do not indicate department or division within the plant or establishment. If accident occurred outside employer's premises at an identifiable address, give that address. If it occurred on a public highway or at any other place which cannot be identified by number and street, please provide place references locating the place of injury as accurately as possible.

10. Place of accident or exposure *(No. and street, city or town, State, and zip code)*

11. Was place of accident or exposure on employer's premises? Yes ☐ No ☐

12. What was the employee doing when injured? *(Be specific. If he was using tools or equipment or handling material, name them and tell what he was doing with them.)*

13. How did the accident occur? *(Describe fully the events which resulted in the injury or occupational illness. Tell what happened and how it happened. Name any objects or substances involved and tell how they were involved. Give full details on all factors which led or contributed to the accident. Use separate sheet for additional space.)*

Occupational Injury or Occupational Illness

14. Describe the injury or illness in detail and indicate the part of body affected. *(E.g., amputation of right index finger at second joint; fracture of ribs; lead poisoning; dermatitis of left hand, etc.)*

15. Name the object or substance which directly injured the employee. *(For example, the machine or thing he struck against or which struck him; the vapor or poison he inhaled or swallowed; the chemical or radiation which irritated his skin; or in cases of strains, hernias, etc., the thing he was lifting, pulling, etc.)*

16. Date of injury or initial diagnosis of occupational illness

17. Did employee die? *(Check one)* Yes ☐ No ☐

Other

18. Name and address of physician

19. If hospitalized, name and address of hospital

Date of report	Prepared by	Official position

OSHA No. 101 (Feb. 1981)

CRITICAL THINKING ACTIVITIES

The dental office in which you are employed is concerned about the cost of medical waste disposal and suggests to you that you should drop off the medical waste at the local pharmacy trash container or the nearby hospital container. What is your reaction to this suggestion?

What are the consequences of not using standard precautions with all patients? For instance, if the following situations presented themselves in your office, what would be your reaction?

a. Why would you feel that you should not use them with a family member?

b. Why would you feel that you should not use them with a young child?

c. Why would you feel that you did not need to use them on a member of the clergy?

18 The Dental Assistant in the Workplace

It is now time to begin a job search. This chapter is really all about you and how you can complete a successful job search. A successful job search requires organization and effort. This chapter provides a myriad of material to aid you in planning and organizing yourself to begin the most important career task of your working life.

When you apply for various jobs, your prospective employers will assume that you have completed your studies and obtained your credentials as a Certified Dental Assistant, a state credential, or certification or degree in business. This chapter emphasizes the tasks necessary to market your skills as a highly educated dental assistant with special training in business office management. Completely read the chapter, and then proceed to answer the questions and complete the materials to prepare you to begin your job search.

LEARNING OUTCOMES

On completion of text and workbook chapters, the student should be able to do the following:
- Define key terms.
- Determine your career goals.
- Identify your personal assets and liabilities for a job.
- Identify legal considerations in hiring.
- Explain the use of preemployment testing.
- Describe new employee orientation.
- Determine desirable characteristics for a job you might seek.
- Determine methods of marketing your skills.
- Identify personal priorities for a potential job.
- Develop a career life philosophy.
- Identify factors to consider in salary negotiations.
- Identify potential areas of employment.
- Prepare data for job applications and interviews.
- Identify potential interview questions.
- List suggestions for a successful interview.
- Prepare an interview follow-up letter.
- Explain how to advance on the job.
- List hints for success in a job on the dental team.
- Describe how to terminate a job.

SHORT-ANSWER OR FILL-IN QUESTIONS

1. Identify five hard skills that a dentist might seek in a dental healthcare employee.

    1. _____

    2. _____

    3. _____

    4. _____

    5. _____

2. What soft skills are desirable in a dental healthcare employee?

_____

_____

_____

3. List 10 desirable characteristics of an administrative assistant.

   1. _____

   2. _____

   3. _____

   4. _____

   5. _____

   6. _____

   7. _____

   8. _____

   9. _____

   10. _____

4. List eight potential job benefits. Which of these would you consider the most important for your personal career?

   1. _____

   2. _____

   3. _____

   4. _____

   5. _____

   6. _____

   7. _____

   8. _____

5. List 10 guidelines for writing a letter of application.

1. _____

2. _____

3. _____

4. _____

5. _____

6. _____

7. _____

8. _____

9. _____

10. _____

6. Discuss the procedure for the following:
   a. Asking for a raise

   _____

   _____

   _____

   _____

   _____

   b. Terminating a job

   _____

   _____

   _____

   _____

   _____

7. List five hints for preparing a résumé.

1. _____

2. _____

3. _____

4. _____

5. _____

MULTIPLE-CHOICE QUESTIONS

8. Which of the following should *not* be included in a résumé?
   a. Emphasis on your qualities and experience
   b. Substantiation of your educational and experience qualifications to justify the abilities that you claim
   c. Being clear and concise in your descriptions
   d. Including a physical description of yourself

9. Which of the following should be included in a résumé?
   a. Health status
   b. Salary information
   c. Educational and experience qualifications
   d. Use of abbreviations or acronyms

10. Which of the following should be avoided during a job interview?
    a. Being prepared to answer a variety of questions
    b. Being too aggressive
    c. Neatness
    d. Accuracy

11. You are offered a job for less money than you had expected based on your experience. Which of the following comments might reflect a positive attitude that you are interested in the job but expect greater compensation?
    a. Really, I can earn more on the other side of town than what you are offering.
    b. I will work for that if that is what you think I am worth.
    c. I am willing to begin for that hourly salary if you will provide me written confirmation that I will be advanced to the salary I am asking within 60 days. I am certain that you will realize my value within that time.
    d. I am willing to begin for that hourly salary, but you are going to have to come up with a big raise in 30 days.

12. Which of the following is *not* the best way to terminate a job?
    a. As soon as you realize that you are unhappy, quit, so you do not have second thoughts.
    b. Give the reason for leaving the job.
    c. Give sufficient notice.
    d. Write a follow-up letter to your verbal resignation.

PRACTICAL ACTIVITIES

13. With two people, have one assume the role of interviewer and the other play the applicant.
    a. Answer the following questions.

Initial Questions

■ How did you learn about this position?

_____

■ What do you know about our practice?

_____

_____

■ Why are you interested in this practice?

_____

_____

■ Tell me about yourself.

_____

_____

_____

_____

■ Why do you think that you are qualified for this position?

_____

_____

■ Describe your most significant accomplishment.

_____

_____

_____

■ What is your definition of "being on time"?

_____

Chapter **18** **The Dental Assistant in the Workplace**

- What qualities are important to you in your work environment?

_____

_____

_____

- If you make a decision and it is questioned, how do you react?

_____

_____

_____

b. Interest in the Job

- Are you currently employed? If so, does your current employer know that you are seeking a new position?

_____

- What would your current employer say makes you most valuable to him or her?

_____

_____

- Why do you want to change jobs?

_____

_____

- What do you consider the ideal job for you?

_____

_____

- What are your long-range and short-range goals?

_____

_____

_____

_____

Education

- What formal education have you had?

_____

- Why did you choose to study dental assisting?

_____

_____

- What was your academic average when you were in school?

_____

- What do you consider your greatest strength? Your greatest weakness?

_____

_____

_____

Experience

- Have you ever been fired or asked to resign from a position?

_____

_____

- Which duties performed in the past have you liked the best? The least? Why?

_____

_____

_____

- Why should I hire you?

_____

_____

_____

- What salary do you expect?

_____

Future on the Job

■ What would you like to know about this practice?

_____

_____

_____

■ Describe how you would demonstrate compassion in this practice.

_____

_____

_____

_____

■ How would you want to integrate into this practice?

_____

_____

_____

_____

■ Discuss six suggestions for success on the job.

1. _____

2. _____

3. _____

4. _____

5. _____

6. _____

14. Write a letter of application for one of the two positions shown in the ads below:

Dental Administrative Assistant needed for a busy orthodontic office. This position requires an energetic, ambitious person who has a broad knowledge of dentistry and business applications. For a person who enjoys a fast pace, this office provides a challenging career opportunity in practice management utilizing modern electronic business systems. Current CDPMA preferred. Write to: Ashley M. Lake, DDS, 611 Main St., SE, Grand Rapids, MI 49502

Dental Administrative Assistant: Interested in an exciting position in a small, professional office? A group dental practice is expanding its clinical facilities. Position demands strong supervisory skills; ability to work effectively under pressure, use good judgment, and accept responsibility; and a working knowledge of OSHA standards. Forward your résumé to: Box #2589, Grand Rapids News, Grand Rapids, MI 49502

Also, prepare a résumé to accompany the letter. Make a copy of the letter and résumé for your personal files. Be selective in the paper on which you print the letter and the résumé because you want to ensure a professional appearance.

For your personal use, review the performance evaluation form in the textbook (Figure 18-10, p. 345). Complete the application form below:

EMPLOYMENT APPLICATION

All information listed on this application will be considered and handled as personal and confidential. Please write or print legibly.

AN EQUAL OPPORTUNITY EMPLOYER

This employer provides equal opportunity to all persons without regard to handicap, race, color, religion, sex, age, or national origin.

Name:			Date of Application:
Address:	City:	State:	Zip:
Home Phone:	Cell Phone:	Social Security Number:	

GENERAL INFORMATION

Position applied for: _____

Available to work: ☐ Full-Time ☐ Part-Time ☐ Temporary

Date available to start work: _____

Are you over 18 yrs. of age? ☐ Yes ☐ No   Will transportation be a problem for you? ☐ Yes ☐ No

If you are not a U.S. Citizen, do you have the right to work in the United States?   ☐ Yes ☐ No

Have you ever been convicted of a felony?   ☐ Yes ☐ No

   (A conviction is not an automatic bar to employment. Each case will be considered on its own merits.)

Does the sight of blood bother you?   ☐ Yes ☐ No

EDUCATION

	Name and address of School	Major/Degree(s)	No. of Years Completed	Did you Graduate?
High School				
Community College				
4 Year Institution				
Vocational				
Other (specify)				

Describe Specialized Training, Apprenticeship, Skills, Seminars, Courses, Extra-Curricular Activities

(Continued)

SKILLS

Task	Circle One		Task	Circle One	
Keyboarding WPM _____	Yes	No	Pour Models	Yes	No
Bookkeeping	Yes	No	Cavitron	Yes	No
Computer Operations	Yes	No	Cast Onlays	Yes	No
Handling Group Insurance	Yes	No	Plaque Control Instruction	Yes	No
Expose, Process, and Mount X-rays	Yes	No	Oral Evacuator	Yes	No
Panoramic X-Rays	Yes	No	Knowledge of Dental Instruments	Yes	No
Have you used insurance software?	Yes	No	Knowledge of Dental Terms	Yes	No
Other: (Describe if yes)					

EMPLOYMENT RECORD

Beginning with your current employer, please list your work experience over the past ten years. You may include pertinent volunteer activities.

Name of Employer		Start Date	End Date
Address	Phone	Start Salary	End Salary
Job Title	Supervisor	Phone	
Duties			
Reason for Leaving			

Name of Employer		Start Date	End Date
Address	Phone	Start Salary	End Salary
Job Title	Supervisor	Phone	
Duties			
Reason for Leaving			

Name of Employer		Start Date	End Date
Address	Phone	Start Salary	End Salary
Job Title	Supervisor	Phone	
Duties			
Reason for Leaving			

REFERENCES

Please provide the name, address, and phone number of at least two non employer/relatives as references.

NAME	ADDRESS	PHONE

EMERGENCY CONTACT

Name	Relationship	
Address	Phone	Alt. Phone

DUTY PERFORMANCE

Are you able to perform the essential duties of the position for which you are applying, either with or without reasonable accommodations?　☐ Yes　☐ No

If yes, please indicate what type(s) of reasonable accommodations are needed:

In the course of making an employment decision, this employer makes it a practice to verify with previous employers information such as dates of employment, description of job duties, attendance records, reason for leaving, etc. If there are any employers you want us to contact, please indicate their names below and reasons why:

_____

_____

_____

_____

I understand that if I am employed and any statement herein is not true, I may be released immediately, I will be paid only through the day of release and this employer may cancel any rights to accrued benefits.

_____　　　　　　_____
　　　　　Date　　　　　　　　　　　　　　　　　　　　Signature

Why is it important to consider a philosophy for work or life? How would this apply to a job interview?